The Healing Shower

Eloise Laws

Copyright 2012 by Eloise Laws and Lake Payne

All rights reserved. No part of this book may be reproduced by any mechanical, photographic, or electronic process, or in the form of a phonographic recording; nor may it be stored in a retrieval system, transmitted, or otherwise be copied for public or private use without written permission from the publisher.

For information regarding permission or additional copies, contact the publisher:

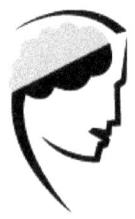

KNOWLEDGE POWER BOOKS
25379 Wayne Mills Place, Suite 131,
Valencia, California 91355
661-513-0308
www.knowledgepowerbooks.com

ISBN: 978-09888644-2-9

Library of Congress Number: Pending

Contributing Writer: Lake Payne
Edited by: Penny Scott
Vocalist: Ywada on "Pink and White
(The Women's Breast Health) Initiative Song"

Cover Design: Juan Roberts, Creative Lunacy
Interior Design: John Sibley, Rock Solid Productions

Printed in the United States of America

This Book Belongs To:

_____

From:

_____

Date:

_____

Table of Contents

Dedication	VIII
Foreword	IX
Inspirational Words	XI
Acknowledgements	XII
Introduction	XIII
My Personal Story	1
The Purpose	11
Fear	15
Action Team...	17
Good Deeds and Services	21
Make a Sign-Up List	
The Preparation	22
Choosing a Shower Coordinator	
Costs and Expenses	
Location	
Keepsake Program	
Acknowledgement Letter	
Invitation List	
Moments to Remember (My Healing Shower)............	25
Letters from Family Members	35
Awards & Recognitions	49

Getting Your House in Order	56
Will/Living Trust	
Power of Attorney/Advanced Health Care Directive	
Recovery ………………………………………………….………….	57
About the Author	59
Recommended Classes/Support Groups	61
Calendar ………………...……….	65
APPENDIX 1 – Power of Attorney Forms (California) …........…..	114
APPENDIX 2 – Advance Health Care Directive Form Instructions…...	121
APPENDIX 3 – Advance Health Care Directive Forms ……....….	126

Dedication

This book is dedicated to the ones we lost to cancer...

Minnie Riperton
Syreeta Wright
Linda Creed
George Duke
Artie Ivie
Mabel Pledger
Hubert Laws, Sr.
Merlin Daggette
D.A McClain
Laura Juanita Brantley Payne
Shirley Ruth Amos
Ella Beatrice Hamilton
Willie Joe Jones
Ron Miller
Robert H. McNeill, Sr.
Goldie Radel
Carmen Cannon Thomas
James "Chuck" Anderson
Kim Dale-Thornton
Beverly Heckstall
Louise Slayton
Arthur L. Slayton, Sr.
Camille Jordan-Slayton

And to all the other Angels watching from above.

Foreword

Let me first begin by expressing the joy I've had knowing Eloise Laws and her husband, Attorney Rickey Ivie for many long years. I knew Rickey from having assisted in his recruitment as a freshman to UCLA. Before that, his brother Artie Ivie (one of the dearly 'remembered'), had given me an invaluable 'thumbs-up,' when I was a freshman at that institution, and much wise counsel as I matriculated. I owe him considerably for helping me to negotiate that maze of 'pitfalls'! Eloise and her siblings have provided me ample enjoyment over many years with their profound talents as purveyors of the best in 'jazz'.

I also had the pleasure of knowing her Memphis connection through certain members of the family's previous generation who resided there, especially the late Erma Laws, another mentor. When I first returned to Los Angeles to do my TV show, "Judge Joe Brown," Èloise and Rickey took me into their home and made me 'feel at home'! I was a member of that "inner circle" she speaks of, and vividly recall the 'chill' when I first heard of her plight.

I also recall the pleasure I received from hearing Eloise tell me what inspired this book, and her vision for helping other cancer patients. Likewise, I'm 'very' flattered with being asked to write this foreword and I do so with profound satisfaction.

Who better than a jazz singer to show you the way to harmonize with yourself in a time of personal physical crisis? Eloise shows a way for your inner, spiritual-self to find rhythm and harmony; to extemporize in a dire theater, crowded with the most raucous of audiences.

You're shown a method and style that brings a positive flow to the cacophony and dissidence of a debilitating illness that assaults with everything; from unwanted permutations of your own cells gone all unruly and wild; all the way through the maelstrom of emotions; storming through you and those who hold you dear.

Eloise guides you melodically through a free-style extemporization allowing, 'you and yours' to join together on the stage she sets, bringing order to the discordance that naturally accompanies the prospect of a looming personal 'extinction-event'. As the lead performer, she sets the flow of the beats and chords, facilitating an adept transformation of despair into a harmonica, stirring resources hidden in the depths of the psyche.

The rhythm she shows us can bring healing to the spirit and is greatly helpful in bringing healing to the body. It is 'stirring'; it is 'moving'! The body and mind are invited into the flow of remission and recovery — those most comforting of prospects — that are so immensely enhanced by her prescription! Everyone — the stricken and those who care — should savor the reverberations of her insight. Eloise gives us a virtuoso performance of mind and body synchronicity; not least through the way she conceptualizes her holistic therapy!

Judge Joe Brown
Emmy Award-Winning Reality TV Judge
TV Show *Judge Joe Brown,* aired 1998 to 2013

Inspirational Words

I first met this beautiful, fiery Scorpio, whom I came to know as Eloise Laws, backstage at the Shrine Auditorium in Los Angeles, California. We were both performers at Danny Bakewell, Jr's Brotherhood Crusade (**www.brotherhoodcrusade.org**), a well-known non-profit organization dedicated to helping disadvantaged communities rebuild and prosper. It was a divine friendship that's lasted more than 25 years. Eloise, a multi-talented, angelic-spirit, possesses vocals which dance among the clouds. Over the years, we established a spiritual bond with the Laws family; i.e. Mother (Miola) Laws, Debra, Hubert, Ronnie, and Blanche. In time, I felt as if I too, was a member of the rhythmic clan.

When I heard the news about Eloise and her plight with breast cancer, my heart dropped. I sensed the immediate connection between Eloise and Syreeta. However, knowing that Eloise is a Scorpio, I knew that she would be the stubborn warrior able to conquer this disease. I'm happy to see that Eloise has written, **The Healing Shower** as a way of not only inspiring others, but also educating those with similar struggles.

As I was reflecting and thinking of Eloise, my song, "Shelter in the Rain," came to mind:

When all the odds say there's no chance,
Amidst the final dance,
I'll be your comfort through your pain
I'll be your shelter in the rain

Stevie Wonder
Grammy award-winning, singer-songwriter, musician, political activist and philanthropist
"Shelter in the Rain" is from Stevie Wonder's 2005 CD titled, *A Time to Love*

Acknowledgements

I want to thank the following people for their love and encouragement:

Rickey, Alexx, Brenda H. Thomas, Mecca Frazier, Lita Gaithers Owens, Debra, Blanche, Donna, Johnny, Hubert, Ronnie, and my dear Mom (Miola Laws). If I've forgotten anyone, please blame it on my head and not my heart. "I love you all."

Eloise

Introduction

This book is written to encourage and uplift all those feeling numb, shock, hopeless, abandoned, without direction, and at death's door. Such emotions are due to an illness that frequently traps patients in darkness searching for the light. But, I honestly believe if a person gets knocked down, it's important to look up. For if you look above, you'll be inspired to rise up. The following account is a testament of how I rose up and made it to the light.

When I first received the life-changing news, I was alone. And, it felt like a lifetime for the technician to get back to me with the results of the second test. I sensed that something was wrong. Then, she appeared and said, "We need to contact your doctor to let him know that we should schedule a biopsy: because of what we found." I just sat there without the ability to move.

MALIGNANT!! I never thought in a million years that my breast would need a biopsy. But, right when the technician said I needed a biopsy: I knew. Deep in my gut, I distinctly knew that I had breast cancer! Within seconds, tears began softly falling from my eyes. Like countless women, this was a fearful time for me and my family.

Following my lumpectomy, I quickly went into survival mode after being told, that this cancer was called DCIS – Ductile Carcinoma in-situ (a non-invasive breast cancer). Meaning that, it had not gone into the milk ducts of my breasts leading to other parts of my body. In essence, I was in Stage 1 of this type of cancer. The physician said that I had a good chance of survival!

He said, "If you're going to have cancer, this is the best cancer to have." I said to him, "You must be kidding! THERE IS NO GOOD CANCER!" Of course, he went on to explain why he made this statement.

Now, I recognized how I was going to survive. And, I was determined to do everything in my power with the assistance of my doctors, family, and friends, to see to it that I achieved such an outcome. Thanks be to God I'm still here!

I was determined to make myself feel good in light of my circumstances. And, as a woman I needed to continue feeling beautiful. So, I went to the spa, had massages, manicures, pedicures, jumped in the Jacuzzi, and sweated like a prune in the sauna. After all of that, I landed in the chair of my hairstylist, Lake Payne. As I sat there, and we thought of how we celebrate life's milestones – weddings, birthdays, anniversaries, and even deaths.

Thus, the idea of **The Healing Shower** was born. We thought, "Why not celebrate this important event in my life, like I do all the others? For, I'm grateful to God for all of the seasons of my life. I should be able to find joy while basking in the sunshine and walking in the rain."

My Personal Story

August 10, 2007, will forever remain a unforgettable day in my life. It was then that my existence took a very dramatic turn. Six months had passed, and it was time for my quarterly mammogram. – You see in 2005, we had been watching the left breast. Therefore, every six months, I routinely examined my left breast. Following the usual procedure, I arrived at my appointment, registered, and changed into a gown.

I was unusually calm that morning. My spiritual mind had already prepared my soul for the imminent news. The first exam was conducted, and I was asked to wait within the holding area. It took some time before the medical technicians and doctors returned, and asked me to come back into the examination room. I was still composed. Not expecting anything bad, but not anything good either. Finally, the nurse and technician said that they would report to my doctor that I would need a biopsy, and that one should be scheduled quickly. Despite the urgency in their voices, I remained cool. No, didn't panic.

Decisions were surfacing only too quickly – retreat to the deep recesses of my mind – the pattern was heavily reminiscent to shooting firecrackers. My thinking was very clear about one element: I was not telling anyone about the report I received that day. Not even my husband was going to hear this news. I wanted to sleep on it and ruminate for a few days. The only fact I did acknowledge was that I was not going to die. This is just a little test of faith.

Instead, I went into denial. My spirit led me to a place where I felt the need to help as many people as possible. I always sensed a desire to assist others, but this condition provoked my heart to move expeditiously. Why? Because deep down in my gut, I believed that my life might be ending. How do I handle this? I just want to be quiet and left alone with my confusion. At some point I had to tell someone. Who will it be first? It had to be someone stronger than me. It had to be a person who would not panic, nor would break down crying in front of me. Who was that person? I prayed and God gave me the answer. Thank God, I am that close to Him (a believer). I told my sister Donna, the baby of our family of eight.

I don't rightly recall exactly how Donna responded or her reactions (See Donna's Letter). I just know it was a tremendous relief to share the news I'd been carrying for hours – even days. After I revealed my condition, the **Healing Shower** was born. Word started spreading rapidly through my immediate family, along with much prayer and comfort. All I can remember during the coming weeks was making sure this news stayed as close to family as possible. A secret. It was my self-preservation taking over. The course that I would take was becoming very clear to me. And, there was no way I could travel this road alone. You think you should, but you can't. With your mind now going 24/7, you need a fairly big, yet tight-knit support system that you can implicitly trust. We formed an "inner circle," where only certain members knew my secret.

Coming from a large family of siblings (sisters) can mean everything. Nonetheless, the real meaning of sisterhood was clear. I would completely turn myself over to Donna. In the meantime, I also told my husband, Rickey, and daughter, Alexx. Rickey said, "My job was to make sure that I could provide you with all the comforts upon needed." I told him in our kitchen and we both held each other and cried. I dropped my head onto his chest and he felt how sad I was. But he was never afraid of the outcome.

Later, Rickey said, "I was sorry you had to lose your breast. But those are the small issues in life." I thought at the time. If I felt less affection and desire as time goes by. I don't know. I've never given it a lot of thought — why I guess I'm afraid to let myself go to that place. – Why? I'm afraid of what I might feel or find. I try not to think about it. I don't. I guess that's best for the marriage and relationship. Rickey's methodical and has envisioned the future.

The Healing Shower

Nevertheless, he affirmed to me that he was by my side for the long haul.

At the same time, as a member of my Action Team (See Action Team), Donna and I maintained contact every hour of the day, planning and gathering information on Breast Cancer doctors, oncologists, reconstructive surgeons, etc. During the quest, another struggle developed: I was growing exhausted. Thus, how would I continue remaining mentally and physically intact health-wise, while making appointments and visits with countless doctors?

After interviewing various doctors, I started feeling comfortable enough to share my cancer outside of my Action Team. I wanted family, extended loved ones, and close friends who were also important business contacts to understand why I had been pushing them away. The floodgates opened concerning who I was consulting for medical care. Everyone wanted to give their advice about what I should and shouldn't be eating. After interviewing numerous doctors, and deciding on the one I would entrust with my situation, I was ready to tackle the world. I became tremendously aggressive about all my duties pertaining to my health. Finally, the serious task of deciding upon my surgery date had become an issue. I wanted to push the date as far back as I could, knowing full well that the sooner I dealt with this matter, the better my position would be in moving past this matter. *(**Special note, I know this is a fearful time, and many of you are like me. You freeze upon hearing your diagnosis. But, please try not to repeat my steps. Be proactive or reactive in the right way. Follow the doctor's advice after getting a second or even third opinion.)* First, the biopsy revealed what stage the breast cancer had traveled. I was very blessed. If you are going to have Breast Cancer, this was the best stage – if that makes sense. It did not at the time, but I later learned my diagnosis meant the cancer had not spread outside the milk ducts. It's called ISC (intraductal spread of carcinoma). We had caught it before it spread outside the breast to other parts of the body. This goes back to if you're going to have Breast Cancer, that's the best one.

However, I feel eternally blessed to have caught this illness early. Ladies, regular breast examinations ladies are crucial!! It means life *or* death. The biopsy revealed the cancer but, a lumpectomy was necessary to see how much breast tissue needed to be removed. Results from the pathology report revealed that more cancer remained in the under the breast tissue. After hearing this report, I was fearful and nervous because I had to make a big decision. Do I have more surgery to peel away tissue, and remain uncertain of whether all of it was removed? Or, have a complete mastectomy and it's all over? In other words, I lose my entire breast, nipple and all! This opens a whole new can of concerns: such as implants, reconstruction, etc. Now, I must return back to the drawing board – more decisions and new information. I decided to have second opinions before I had my surgery. (*I suggest you do likewise if you find yourself in similar circumstances*).

It was exciting interviewing doctors and learning so much about a complex subject. I never imagined I would have to explore this topic for my own survival! Then again, never know what life has to offer down the road. One thing is for sure, I knew I had to remain open to all opinions. During this time, **Healing Shower** came into fruition while looking ahead of my future and having dialogue with all of the medical professionals and family members. I along with my friend and hairstylist, Lake collaborated ideas. We started talking about how important it is for friends and family members to understand what you're feeling, and the type of support needed, while undergoing treatment for various forms of cancer.

The idea was to productively involve loved ones during hospital and/or home recovery. I created a Good Deeds and Services/Sign-Up List, encouraging the need for cooking, cleaning/bathing the patient, running errands, updating medical records, helping patient with bathroom duties, note-taking for all medical appointments, feeding the dog, and answering phones. A lot of these duties remove a heavy burden from the patient.

The Healing Shower

The *Healing Shower* occurs before the surgery – a few days or weeks, if possible. Planning it can be very exciting. Holding it is a lot fun and spiritually uplifting.

<u>Discerning Clarity</u>

I took two days before the reconstruction surgery to meditate. There were times during the day when I stopped to talk to myself and pray. This was very relaxing, as well as building faith, confidence and courage. It's not easy to know that you are putting yourself into the hands of total strangers. Although these people are trained professionals, you don't know them personally. Nor, do you know or have any idea what kind of night these surgeons had before they arrived in the anesthesiology and operating room prior to prepping and putting you into the unconscious state you must enter before your surgery takes place and becomes successful.

Of course, I am a strong believer in prayer and faith (i.e. God). So, I concentrated all of my energy and focused intensely upon a divine connection, in order to receive a (timely) supernatural intercession. My desire was not entirely inspired by totally selfish intentions, but encapsulated a selfless one as well.

I was vastly successful due to the fact that I had a lot of help and steadfast support from both family and friends. I had two prayer warriors who came to pray with me the day before my surgery. We prayed for one solid hour. I guess you could say we prayed and didn't stop until we got a clear answer from God Almighty. We made our connection. It was a beautiful shedding of negativity. The rest of my day was very peaceful and positively optimistic. Five thirty a.m. on Friday, March 7, I reported to admissions at Cedars-Sinai Hospital in Los Angeles, Calif. We were punctual. I had my Action Team with me; my mom, Miola, the most important supporter; my husband, Rickey, and daughter, Alexx, of course. I was also surrounded by all of my sisters; Blanche, Donna and Debra. On my husband's side of the family, there was his aunt, Merlin

Eloise Laws

Daggett (now deceased), his aunt's daughter, Georgette Daggett, and his sister-in-law, Sylvia Drew Ivie. My very best friend, Brenda Brown Thomas of 44 years, flew in from Baltimore, Maryland (she is a minister and close confidant). Pastor Fuller was also present, which was comforting and considerate since it was five-thirty in the morning! And, last but certainly not least, was my Heavenly Father, who was present. And, the only one who actually had access to my whereabouts, while the surgery was being performed.

Can you believe the surgery took nine and one-half hours? I am here and writing this book to say, "Thank you," Heavenly Father. Amen.

Having an Action Team is not just important, it's everything. The morning went like clockwork. We prayed, laughed, and talked right up to the time I went into the room for surgery.

The surgeons were: Dr. David Femiliar, who removed the cancer and Dr. Marvin Slate, who performed the reconstruction. I know that God was in control and in the room because the anesthesiologist approached me with an enormous smile on his face. I was the first in the surgery pool that morning at 6:30 a.m. It was fun and I had a certain resolve watching the marked place (i.e. preparation room for surgery) come alive slowly. By the time I was prepped for the surgery, paperwork, marking of my body for my reconstruction surgery. I was ready. Accompanied by my "dream team," I was more than prepared. After meeting everyone who would actually assist in the surgery room, my enthusiasm was confidently reinforced. I was told, "We would like for you to sing for us before we put you to sleep." I laughed and sang a verse of, "How Great Thou Art." The next thing I knew, I was being awakened in the recovery room. I thanked God right away that I had made it through to the next level – recovery. Both surgeons were in the recovery room when I awakened. I remained there for hours at least until a room was ready for my occupancy. In the meantime, I did experience an uneasy recovery. Nausea was the order of the day. It was an unfortunate side-effect of the anesthesia. This remained with me for at least eight to nine hours post-surgery. It was a true test of my faith because I refused to take the anti-nausea medication. I took this position because with the first surgery of the mastectomy they administered anti-nausea meds automatically, and I had a terrible negative reaction. I couldn't remember the name of that particular medication and they didn't have a record. So, my decision was to wait and suffer it out.* *This goes back to my suggestion of keeping a personal medical journal of meds and experiences in the hospital.* I survived. I was told I was not a nice person during this time. So, I spent the next day apologizing to all.

<u>To God Be the Glory</u>

    I spent four nights in Cedars-Sinai Hospital, which the administrators took great care to ensure my needs were met. And when the time arrived for me to leave, I was taught how to care for the tubes that were still attached to my breast. These spouts required draining for at least ten days. The additional preparation was needed for breast reconstruction surgery scheduled for about four months later.

    The protocol goals I tried to set at this point seemed cruel, downright unjustly, unachievable. I still felt very inadequate. I knew I had a long, long road ahead. This trial made me well aware that I had begun my inexorable march into the enemy's territory (region). I intended to make it a slow march. Any other way would be setting myself up for possible failure. The Action Team will be on patrol, and they will prop me up when I commence to lean or fall.

    This is the importance of finding a support group (See Support Group/Classes Section) outside of your family and team. You have the opportunity to meet and dialogue with women and men who share similar aspirations, attitudes, fears, inadequacies, and possibly depression. There will be days when you "feel down and alone," and desire to be left alone with yourself and your thoughts. In the early stages of cancer, some are unable to physically rise out of bed or the house because they don't have the strength. Many say it's either physically or spiritually exhausting. I can attest to those emotions. Everything becomes still — life seems to dramatically slow down. Maybe, that is good because in order to heal, I believe it's God's way of getting your attention. <u>Slow it down</u>

When I was made to go to the final stage and undergo a mastectomy (took me out of my comfort zone), I did not want to face any of it. I felt like a woman with cancer being stripped of her womanhood. Even though you give me replacement breast, and that's a personal choice — something greater has been lost—what you were born with has been taken away. A woman's breasts are like her hair. They're her crown and glory. For me, I had the most beautiful body. My breasts were round and plump. I don't feel sexy in that way anymore. How do you get that back? It took time to feel way.

<u>Supernatural Whispers to My Soul</u>

What made me change my mind from only having one breast removed as opposed to both? My best friend, Brenda, from Baltimore was in the waiting room with me before I was taken into surgery. Brenda quietly sequestered me away from the crowd and asked, "Why are you removing both breasts?" She went on to state, "I know it's not a good time to bring this up, since you are already scheduled to have a total mastectomy. But, a higher source is putting in my heart to tell you not to remove both breasts, if you don't have to."

Shortly after, that they called me in to prep me for the surgery. Once inside, the nurses and leading surgeon, Dr. David Femiliar, came in to speak with me to see if I was ready for the procedure. Dr. Slate entered and measured me for the reconstruction phase after the main surgery. I felt compelled to open up and ask him while it was fresh on my mind. I asked, "Do you think I should have both breasts removed?" He answered, "Do you have cancer in the other breast?" I said, "No, but everyone involved such as

The Healing Shower

Dr. Femiliar and my family recommends I remove the other breast as a precautionary measure: for not getting cancer in the opposite Breast."

The Lord spoke through my best friend, Brenda. My best friend of 44 years and prayer partner, Brenda knew that having a total mastectomy was a heavy burden on my heart. God interceded. Nevertheless, Dr. Femiliar was quite annoyed, as well as confused. Removing two breasts is far less expensive and requires different paperwork from the administration and insurance office for billing purposes. But, I highly doubt those are reasons for his irritation. You see, we had spent months deciding and going over this step-by-step: All the details, top-to-bottom, for months. So, naturally he and his team of medical staff were prepared for the full "Monty."

Of course there was much delay with going ahead with the surgery because all the paperwork had to be changed from the entry/administrative office right up to the surgery preparatory room. With a procedure of this kind at a major hospital a lot of paperwork is involved. Always go with your emotions regarding life-changing issues. I made the right decision after listening to the small DIVINE whispers within my psyche and soul. It only took seconds to internalize then verbalize this pertinent recommendation originating from the immaterial into the material world.

Only a few of my Action Team members were informed of my decision until after the surgery.

The Purpose

What is a Healing Shower? In actuality, the first question posed should be: What is the importance of rituals in modern-day society? Why do we believe the **Healing Shower** is important for your family? It allows each family member an opportunity to receive and give their total input on what to do in case of the unexpected. No one knows what the future may entail. The **Healing Shower** assists in awakening your senses regarding what the patient will have to experience during his or her illness: surgery, pneumonia, accident and/or extended hospital stay. This is a time for loved ones to come together and celebrate positive energy before a loved one goes off to face an intensive surgery, i.e. cancer.

It's the opportune time to wish this person well on a safe and healthy road to recovery. All too often, a person enters into surgery and/or death alone and is too afraid to express emotions welling up inside of her – fear, sadness, anxiety, rage, helplessness, defeat, failure, et cetera. As a result, she ends up separating herself from the people she needs the most – family and friends. Enter the **Healing Shower**. We have designed this ritual to be a celebration and time of happiness.

A **Healing Shower** provides an individual with the preparation required to confront and conquer the illness that has invaded her life and personal space. During this shower, loved ones are encouraged to sing, perform spoken word/poetry, or offer kind words of encouragement. This is also a place of forgiveness for old grudges. Weight can be lifted off one's shoulders when peace is resolved. With respect to the Deeds and Services/Sign-Up List (See Action Team), guests can publicly offer their services. Loved ones will be held more accountable when saying what they will do in front of others, as opposed to simply writing it down. Family and friends can also have open dialogue about cancer with the patient. Hopefully, all with an understanding that this event not only helps one person, but the collective group participating as a team!

The bottom line is this: when a serious illness strikes, it will unfold regardless of whether or not one is ready! Why not be as prepared as possible to face what lies ahead? Through this process, loved ones flank the sides of the patient to offer guidance, unconditional love, support, words of wisdom, shared tears, a sense of community, and unity during this very difficult time.

Consequently, she becomes empowered because she's equipped not only with the physical bond provided by her network of friends and family members, but also equipped with an emotional armor of strengthening tools and techniques received during her celebratory event. Hospital visitation rules should also be established and communicated amongst your community of friends and family. This plays a major role in the patient's wellness and recovery. Although there are visiting hours printed, one should always call before coming to see the patient. This allows the patient if they she is resting or sleeping to continue to do so.

Don't forget she is in the hospital and doctors and nurses are constantly in and out of her room; conducting tests; drawing blood; or doing something as simple as changing the bedding; and maybe giving a sponge bath. All of these duties occur while one is in the hospital for long periods of time. You must be cognizant of all these possibilities before visiting your friend or relative, while she is recovering in the hospital. Very Important!!

She is in an extremely sterile environment. So, before you enter her space, it is very important that you wash your hands before embracing the patient. Remember, she is susceptible to all kinds of outside germs. Her body is in a weakened state. She is there to heal, survive and go home. Call to make sure the patient is able and can tolerate, or desire to have visitors. Most people are under the impression because you are in the hospital you are confined, locked up and want company. The real reason you are there is to heal

The Healing Shower

and recover (get well). You would rather be home if you had your choice. Sadly, I think many assume you are on your deathbed, and are happy that they took the time to come and visit.

However, there are countless jobs friends could handle for you that would be far more productive. For instance, writing a "Thank You" note, for the beautiful flowers you've been receiving while in the hospital. Also, picking up and sorting your mail, for when you are ready to deal with it. Checking to see what needs to be done at your home while you're away is another helpful duty. The ***Healing Shower*** encourages and provides instruction for all of these services.

Faith is taking the first step even when you don't see the whole staircase.
Dr. Martin Luther King, Jr.

The Healing Shower

Fear is nothing, the real thing is courage.
- Ndebele proverb

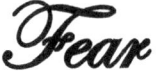

Fear is a traitor. We must face our demons sooner rather than later, or they will take over and destroy our lives. If you have a problem, an illness, or whatever in life – you must attend to it or it will attend to you in an extremely negative way. I find that if you can walk, then you can also run. But, you must first put it in your consciousness. It then manifests a plan. Put fear into action. So, it's the same with a serious illness such as *cancer*. Be it breast, colon, cervical, stomach or all the others – tackle it head on!

If you don't deal with it, that situation will deal with you, and the outcome will surely be death. Fortunately, it doesn't have to end that way. You must be proactive immediately upon finding out. I have a friend who's been diagnosed with Breast Cancer. Because of fears, she will not get treated but thinks she can pray it away. Yes, prayer is very necessary and so is faith, along with that you need to treat the symptoms medically. And, prayer without works is futile. She has two choices; she can treat the cancer or she can die. Life is too short to wake up one day with regrets: or, not wake up at all. God never said, "Life would be easy." He just promised that life would be worth the struggle. You are in it to **WIN**, and **WIN** you must!

My girlfriend who has this fear is using High Blood Pressure medication as an excuse. The technicians, surgeons and nurses said her blood pressure is too high for the surgery. She refuses to take the High Blood Pressure medication because she and a friend believe that it will cause a deadly side-affect. So, it's a Catch-22 situation – damned if you do, and damned if you don't! She passed the physical exam with the exception of High Blood Pressure. As we know this poses a danger when being put under anesthesia. Therefore, she chose to not remove the *Cancer* from her Breast. **Fear**. She is going to wait and see what happens. Most people do that and then it's too late. The cancer has spread throughout the body by then. You lose. It's all over, but the crying remains.

God provides you the will and strength to reach down inside, unlocking your inner courage. Trust me, if I can do it, you can – anyone can. Be thankful for the bad things in life, for they open your eyes to the good things you weren't acknowledging before the situation occurred. Our greatest weakness lies in giving up. The most certain way to succeed always is to make one more attempt. Leave fears in the dust and run all the way to the finish line! Remember, fear is not a friend, but your enemy. <u>Deal with it</u>. This is war. This fight against cancer must be fought with every being of your body – you are on the battlefield!

The Healing Shower

ACTION TEAM

One of the first things you need to do in being proactive toward your recovery is create an Action Team. This consists of family, friends, casual acquaintances, community/religious leaders, and medical support staff. The main objective of this team is to guide and assist the patient on her/his journey. These people are there to help you every step of the way. Remember this isn't a quest you should take alone. Loneliness can make the process more difficult to handle. Opening yourself up for others to assist is part of the process. It humbles you because you have to allow others to help.
You become the GPS, while the Action Team drives.
Once you pick a solid group of people for the Action Team, start to write down a list of things that need to take place. It can be anything, including making dinner, sending off bills, and notifying others of this new process. The whole point of this task is to figure out what help is required so your mind will be at ease. Oftentimes, many like to help out, but can't because they don't know what type of assistance you need. This will also eliminate wasted time. After you have created a Good Deeds and Services/Sign-Up List (See below), evaluate your Action Team, and start assigning duties.
Some of the things you will need help with are hospital trips and recovery. Pick at least three (3) people. Why three? Most people have the same individual with them day in and day out. That helper sometimes starts becoming drained, resentful, and controlling. The reason why is because you have given them a huge job that requires numerous individuals. This is another reason why some people become discouraged when assisting others. They don't want enormous responsibility. By limiting the number of helpers, you can distribute the duties and remain in control.
Try to see if anyone in the family has a medical background. My sister was a tremendous help at my visits. I felt like I understood visitations much better when was present at my appointments: versus in the beginning when I was going to the appointments alone. Find a

good note taker. You want to make sure to keep a journal throughout the whole process. Information that the doctors provide is important, but also after the surgery, you will need to note any adverse reactions from the medication. Look for a nurturer. This will be the one to hold your hand in the midst of an emotional breakdown. It's best to have a comforter that offers big hugs and tells you everything will be OK. This is a person that has dealt with lots of tragic situations, and can be very optimistic. Remember, these are *examples* of different attributes of people that can be very helpful to you. Also consider a/an:

- **Confidant** - knows how you're feeling, and your deepest, darkest secrets. She/he listens without judgment.

- **Informant** - sends out your Medical Press Release(s) (for the sake of a fancy name). Informs family circle of what you want them to know. Provides updates either on the telephone, email, or Social Media pages.

- **Strong Medical Team** - Their bedside manners are vitally important. My team treated me like a friend. This helps tremendously with the recovery process. Share some of your personal interests in life to your medical team. In this way, your medical team will know more about you.

- **Spiritual Advisor** – has a spiritual or metaphysical background. He or she will help you channel positive thoughts and will facilitate the healing shower. He can help you tackle the illness from a spiritual perspective. Illness in my opinion can sometimes enter our lives for various reasons. One main motive is stress. Oftentimes, we hold so much stress within our bodies that it builds up rock-like cells. We may be holding on to some grudges that we haven't released.

The **Hèaling Shower** is the place to find forgiveness, which allows you to be healed. "Stress Kills" can only be a true statement if you allow it. How often do people say the cause of death was really due to stress? In my opinion, stress creates the disease. Then, the worry over the disease, instead of getting to the core of the problem is what kills us. This is the time to dig deep and see if there is anything bothering you in life. Reflect on your childhood. It's time to find closure. Let this be the opportunity to not only heal from cancer, but other burdens that may be haunting you. This shower is a cleansing of the mind, body and soul. Each drop of water represents a person showering his or her love upon you, assisting in your road to recovery.

Post sign-in sheets with two-hour intervals, and leave open opportunities for loved ones to occasionally bring lunch from your favorite restaurants. Don't be afraid to let people know that you also accept monetary donations (everything helps). Additional miscellaneous items may include feeding the dog or cat. Someone might be in charge of ensuring you have fresh flowers. Another can drop by and read Daily Bread/Affirmations to you. Make your home a sanctuary, instead of a place for friends and family to catch up, while you're trying to recover.

Eloise Laws

GOOD DEEDS and SERVICES – MAKE a SIGN-UP LIST

The *Healing Shower* is a Rite of Passage for individuals faced with tragic, life-altering illnesses. Beginning with the diagnosis, the patient, her family and friends start planning for her walk down an uncharted road. To prepare for this journey, several items need to be in place. Here is a list of suggested tasks, people can agree to the following;

1. **24-hour Companion and Confidant** (In-Home Help (IHH) – this person should have an incredible flexible schedule, as in certain cases a patient isn't capable of being alone.
2. **Schedule Medical Appointment** – keep Medical Records up to date. Maintain Copies of all Medical Records.
3. **Collect Mail**.
4. **Meal Preparation** – for Family members, as well as for the patient when she returns home from the hospital.
5. **Grocery Shop**
6. **Pay Bills** – ensure Medical Bills are especially confronted.
7. **Monitor Hospital and Home Visits** – ensure
8. visits don't become <u>overwhelming</u> for the patient (while in the hospital, as well as at home recuperating).
9. **Run Errands**.
10. **House Clean** – help patient and/or family maintain order of home until patient recovers.
11. **Bathe and Clean/Bathroom Clean-Up Detail.** (Assist the Patient in going to the restroom, as well as taking baths and/or showers.)
12. **Commit to Drive Patient to all Return Medical Visits** (multiple people).

The Healing Shower

13. **Dispense and Administer Medication** – sign on to assist with Medication Therapy (as needed).
14. **Receive and Return Phone Calls/Messages** – to be handled later by patient.
15. **Note-taker at Doctor/Therapy Appointments** – for all important information.
16. **Write/Mail** "Thank You" notes.
17. **Schedule Personal Beauty Care Appointments**.

*If you don't have a relative, friend and/or neighbor to help with these Deeds/Services, contact County Services and ask for IHH Services, which are covered based on special needs.

** One purpose of the shower is to make sure the patient is completely worry-free of all obligations during her recovery and healing time.

Eloise Laws

THE PREPARATION

Choosing a Shower Coordinator

This should be someone who has a flexible schedule. The facilitator is responsible for making the day come together. Some of his/her duties include; assisting with creating the guest list; working with the honoree for planning the shower; sending out the Acknowledgement Letter and Invitations; and helping to develop a registry of the healing items you may need such as the physical chores we mentioned earlier. Books with affirmations and holistic products are always nice.

Costs and Expenses

While we do want to keep costs at a minimum, please ensure that the focus of the shower remains on health, family, friends and love. Also, my theme surrounded the acronym for H.E.A.L, which concentrates on "**H**" for **hope**; **E** represents the word "**educate**"; "**A**" was symbolic for "**affirmation**"; and "**L**" signified "**liberate yourself**." Thus, certain party and craft stores, as well as religious boutiques, may have a plethora of supplies.

Location

The facility should be a place that brings the patient comfort and a sense of security. In general, this is ideally her home but if she happens to already be hospitalized, consider a lounge in the hospital.

Keepsake Program

Aside from any photography or videotaping that may occur, you might want to create and distribute a keepsake program. Consider the heading for my program: ***Healing Shower, a***

The Healing Shower

refreshing for the mind, body and spirit (See attachment). Include the moderator's name, definition of the acronym for H.E.A.L. This is merely a guideline, and specific to my circumstances. Select words symbolic of your lifestyle and that are meaningful to your family.

Acknowledgement Letter

Allow your Acknowledgement Letter as the prime opportunity, and formal way of informing people about the reason for the gathering, as well as an invitation of commitment to participate with the patient on this quest to become cancer-free! All interested participants will RSVP to attend an intimate healing event. This letter can act as a safe way to inform people of the illness, and see that life within itself is a celebration.

This invitation also informs individuals straight from the "horse's mouth." Stories can be switched around when it's word-of-mouth. However, this Acknowledgement Letter allows you to take ownership of the cancer, which you will soon set free. It doesn't want to be there. In writing the letter, you will automatically feel relief, as a burden is being released from your shoulders.

You play a major role before anything can be expected of the doctors. Rise above the circumstance at-hand. Share this information with people who care about you. Make a choice to add the *Healing Shower* invitation along with the Acknowledgement Letter. Or, create and send an invitation separately. Guests will appreciate the fact that you took the time to inform them in a formal way regarding something that usually has a negative connotation. This letter also assists your small village in serving you. The purpose is to gather together those that can be helpful in your healing process. There is a story that needs to unfold and hopefully through the actual ceremony some wonderful things will take place.

Also, take this opportunity to ask for prayer. I truly believe in the power of prayer, and the more people you have praying, the better. Incidentally, this movement of prayer jumpstarts the

Eloise Laws

Healing Shower method! Cancer is no different from anything else in your life that you feel doesn't serve you. That's the way you have to think of it. When we are happy, harmful experiences don't exist. Therefore, your Acknowledgement Letter is the building block upon which your family and friends (fans) use to guide how they will support and cheer you on throughout your toughest days. Within this letter, include a Good Deeds and Services/Sign-Up List, along with a Registry of items from a Health food store. Then, you can do a separate shower invitation for the actual event, if you prefer.

Invitation List

Who should be invited to this life-changing event held in your honor? Dependable, reliable and flexible persons with a daily schedule that's adjustable because <u>reliability</u> is the key. I was precise with respect to my guest list, ensuring that only family and close friends held dear to my heart were invited. Remember, this is one of the most important moments in your life! It's just as momentous as a wedding day, the birth of a child, et cetera. It's my opinion that the bigger the shower, the more distractions, leading to the loss of focus and real meaning of the shower. (This also helps control the flow of positivity within your event.)

Allow yourself time to discuss forgiveness with loved ones. Forgiveness brings new life. Unresolved grudges brings suffering and bondage. The healing shower can rinse your soul from pain but only if you allow it.

The human body experiences a powerful gravitational pull in the direction of hope. That is why the patient's hopes are the physician's secret weapon. They are the hidden ingredients in any prescription.
- **Norman Cousins**

Moments to Remember
(My Healing Shower)

The sun was setting as roughly 20 people gathered at my home for what would be an unforgettable occasion. Growing up in a family of eight children, this shower could've easily turned into a gigantic bash. However, today was not about the quantity it was strictly about the quality. More importantly, it was about my long-term recovery and healing that was at stake! My pastor, Perry Fuller, agreed to facilitate the event. You might also want a Spiritual Advisor, minster, or close friend to direct your ***Healing Shower***. Some churches even have trained practitioners for these types of events.

Chairs were arranged in a ring, representing a *healing circle*. They surrounded my seat in the middle, symbolizing completeness. Because I held an evening shower, I combined natural light with candles lit throughout the living room. All showers should create a warm, relaxing environment with soft, contemplative, smooth jazz or classical music playing in the background as guests arrive. I chose contemplative music. Try to construct a soothing, spa-like ambiance for your event.

Thirst-quenching, flavorful drinks such as cucumber water and fresh lemonade were some of the beverages provided. As this is a spiritual gathering, I <u>DO NOT</u> recommend serving alcohol prior to the beginning of your ***Healing Shower***. I also advise that your participants' minds be *spiritually focused*, and ready to receive from a Higher Power. We actually formed an inseparable healing circle, emotionally rotating on the axis of love.

Did I like sitting in the center of this healing circle? Sure, I adored being the center of attention. However, I wasn't singing or acting. My family and friends gathered around me to support me in the toughest battle of my life! I was terrified and facing the unknown! I don't like being in unknown territory. Thankfully, a circle of love surrounded me – a sign that my show must go on. I took a deep breath and closed my eyes.

Pastor Fuller started the event with an Opening Prayer, and then we sang, "Amazing Grace." During the Welcome and Purpose, the pastor said he was facilitating in order to promote happy feelings. Pastor Fuller is extremely dedicated, and has been present at my bedside to pray with me and my family throughout the course of my surgeries and recovery. He provided the definition for the acronym of "heal," or **H.E.A.L.** Whereas **"H"** represented *hope*; **"E"** signified *educate*; **"A"** meant *affirmation*; and **"L"** symbolized the empowering meaning of *"liberate yourself."*

Yes!! Those were extremely powerful concepts chosen for my journey. Yet, everyone bravely embraced each word, sharing their love and responsibilities for this next part of my life-changing quest. Considering the letter **"H,"** it was our *hope* that I was going to be healed. Hope means the best is yet to come. We all desire to have more in our lives, but are we willing to endure excruciating trials in order to receive an outstanding outcome?

Clearly, I was at everyone's mercy and all I could do was hope for the best. I was hoping for: a successful recovery; smooth transition; and clarity as to why I was facing a traumatic experience. Yes, I said it! This has not been easy. My life as I know it was about to change with a part of my body becoming permanently altered. THAT'S SCARY!! I know I shouldn't be afraid, but I am. When we change from teens to adults, we don't give it a second thought. Let's face it. This is different, and I found myself treading in unfamiliar territory. Pastor Fuller led us through a few mantras beginning with the words offering hope, "I believe…." As for me, I believe that I have countless accomplishments that I'm in the process of fulfilling!

The Healing Shower

My hope increased after each attendee affirmed what hope meant, and how he/she could use hope to help support my recovery. I was very fortunate during the healing shower to be in the presence of two magnificent women. One is my mother, Miola, and the other is my aunt, Elizabeth. Both of these women are in their 90s, and their spirits light up any room. We transformed into a "wisdom circle" when it was time to focus on the letter "**E**" as in "*educate*."

Pastor Fuller said that it was not only crucial that we are all educated about caring for someone recovering from surgery, but also knowledgeable about the causes of cancer, in general. Incidentally, before being diagnosed with breast cancer, I'd been faithfully supporting the Neal Bogart Foundation. This organization supports children with cancer. More than 13,000 kids die of complications from cancer annually. I continue to support them as much as possible by purchasing tickets for their annual luncheon.

Lake and I joined my Action Team after I revealed to her my breast cancer diagnosis. She told me about her client, D.A., who was about my age and also had a daughter the same age as my daughter, Alexx. Unfortunately, D.A. passed away. But Lake thought creating the ***Healing Shower*** was a good idea. I had already discussed this with my youngest sister Donna. By this time, my Action Team was slowly coming forming.

I met Lake on a photo shoot for my album cover, and that day I had no idea she would become so relevant in my life. Lake was an open book – always ready to learn as well as give information that she'd learned over the years. I knew with her on my side, there would never be a "bad hair day." Shelly Fisher was another interesting relationship. She was a person that I met from a mutual friend by the name of Ron Miller. He was a gifted songwriter and producer, who wrote amazing Top 10 hits including, "For Once in My Life," "Yester-Me, Yester-You, Yesterday," "Touch Me in the Morning," "Put Me On," and "If I Could." Ron was a wonderful and dear friend who passed away in 2007 of **cardiac arrest**, after suffering from a long battle with **emphysema** and **cancer**. Again, we must educate our loved ones on all the causes of cancer to save our families.

Shelly also had admiration for me as an artist. She was a financial advisor, as well as a singer, so she understood the difficulty of being successful in the music industry. Over the years we crossed paths and remained in contact. Shelly was always someone that you could usually rely upon. But this day, she stepped up to the occasion. She wrote a song called, "The Healing Shower." That was such a glorious gift to share, as well as extend her helping hand. Once again, it confirmed to me that the relationship that started off as social and casual had evolved into something much greater. I was starting to get it. This healing shower was helping me pay attention o very important elements of life.

The rate of minority women diagnosed with breast cancer continues to rise at an astonishing rate. So, we need to be proactive in checking ourselves, and informing our loved ones. Once you educate yourself about a situation and do your part then the fear slowly disappears. And each one vowed to teach one about the dangers of breast cancer.

With respect to the letter "**A**," Lake blessed us with spoken word, and then Pastor Fuller defined the concept of "*affirmation.*" My husband Rickey was the first in the family to speak. He affirmed that the love he had for me was stronger than ever before, and that he would support me throughout the whole process. He vowed to be the shoulder of strength to carry me on. He said he wasn't going anywhere. It was then, that I came to realize that this cancer was not going to affect the love that Rickey and I have for one another.

This cancer isn't stronger than the love we have, and through our love we will overcome this experience together. I was in tears as Rickey expressed his profound love for me. It was very different from the vows on our wedding day. I needed to *affirm* every day that I was going to be in perfect health. My life is going to be OK, and I'm going to beat cancer! These words were coming from a transformed place and it felt good. I needed to hear that.

The Healing Shower

Right after my husband, my daughter, Alexx stood up and gave me the biggest hug. She told me how much she loved me. Rickey and Alexx had been very silent up until this point. So, I didn't know how they were feeling during the whole process. And the question came up in my mind if they were okay. After that, a ripple effect was created. Everyone in the circle stood up and embraced me with hugs and shared their love for me. I felt like relationships had been mended.

Our Lord's Prayer resonated in my mind, "Forgive our debts as we forgive our debtors." Resentment that might have occurred at any point in my life with any person in the room had been forgiven. Old grudges and deep-rooted pain in my life had been restored. I was in a form of true completion. The love I expressed for myself was being reciprocated.

On this journey called life, our faith and beliefs will be tested. I affirmed that I am worthy of experiencing more love in my life than pain. The road that we're on isn't perfect. There will be flooded streets, accidents, detours, and bumps, causing me to slow down. Maybe, we need those occasional thumps to refocus our thoughts, and return to being closer to God. He always says, "When you are down is when you will call on Him the most. And, and your sense of faith will truly be tested." More importantly, this shower made me understand I had unresolved issues in my life, and needed clarity before I expected the doctors to perform their magic. Affirm that Plan A is all you need and it will work.

Use your power of the tongue, which can declare life or death into a situation. Think of children, and how they come from a place of knowing. We were once those same kids. Adulthood has brought many fears and insecurities into unwarranted situations. Unfortunately, we have forgotten the power bestowed upon us by our Almighty Creator! I suggest you pray and develop similar positive motivational phrases or mantras. Beginning with "I Am… I Am. A perfect gem truly blessed to be in great health." The key is once you affirm it, you have to own it and believe it. If you choose to bring a doubtful thought behind the affirmation, you will cancel out your positive thought because of the negative energy.

Pastor Fuller said it's important to understand the significance of maintaining a positive outlook about your health, and how it *affirms* your position in the universe. He confirmed to me that everyone has a path to walk in life, and this is the path that has been destined for me. I am walking on the correct path.

When we focused on the letter "**L**," which represented "*liberate yourself,*" the concept was led by a dance movement. The dancer moved gracefully, soaring and flowing – free like a bird. I too, was going to be soaring – free of this cancer. No more poison would be *invading* my body. This disease had no right to hold me hostage. Liberate yourself! It's time to break free from cancer! We are here to live to the fullest. I am fighting for a better life – an upgrade from life, as I knew it to be when I was **LIBERATED** before this cancer entered my body. This experience alone is making me wiser. I am looking at things from a whole new perspective. Just hearing the way people think about me made me reevaluate how I thought of myself.

I have been taking myself for granted and you shouldn't do that. We all need to step back and appreciate who we are on both the human side, as well as our spiritual aspect. Throughout the day, the only thing most of us think about is the stress of acquiring material things: how we don't have enough money to gain them, or the concerns of the accomplishments our kids will achieve.

On this day, **"L"** also embodied an outpouring of *love* in the highest power. It is one of the possessions we can't live without, but for some reason we don't acknowledge love enough in our lives. Nor do we demonstrate it to those who we care for. If you don't love your job, you will search for another position. Lack of love in a relationship can lead to a divorce. Love for the game wins championships. Now it's my turn. I must love life more than life itself. Loving life is giving the highest praise to the Creator of life. Some moms ensure their kids are well-maintained. However, when

The Healing Shower

the tables are turned, those same mothers neglect their own appearance, and everything else that pertains to their presence. Our daily focus is *lack* instead of *prosperity* and *abundance*. Clearly, it was time to let myself know how much I was in love with myself. This body has been running strong for many years. I can't say I made all of my scheduled tune-ups or oil change appointments. I admit. There have been plenty of times I have driven myself on **E**. No more!

Finally, I'm seizing the fact that life is actually a blessing and understanding the importance of life. Being an entertainer, I am always faced with the perception of my image. Now, I have to deal with an image alteration that definitely ain't Botox. My body was going to be different. Plus, I was going to be off my feet, while undergoing the recovery process. What was that going to be like? Would my husband be able to cope? I was always "put together." Being laid up in the bed was something that was not Eloise – the award-winning recording artist – the actress – the Tony-nominated performer! This was part of the unknown effects of cancer that haunts us. Can cancer affect my marriage? These are the types of variables you contemplate, and it can create high-stress levels in your life. Circumstances are going to be different, and change will either be good or bad. Luckily, I had the power of the **Healing Shower**. Yes, I vowed to become cancer-free. I had cancer, but it did not have me!

During this moment of reflection on the phrase, "liberate yourself," something that remains unforgettable was my when younger sister Debra (Laws) came forward to perform. She stood up, and my goodness, it sent chills up my spine! We had experienced so much together. Debra and I have sung together for many years. She's had Top 10 R&B hits for the songs "Very Special," "Be Yourself," and "Meant for You." There was never a time when I thought she wouldn't be around, and I knew she felt the same way about me. She performed the Dolly Parton hit, "I Hope You Dance." My God!! That girl can sing!! Her voice filled the room. Tears welled up in her eyes as the words of the song came out of her mouth.

Angelic is all I have to say. The tears came but they we not tears of sadness or sorrow: These were tears of happiness. Joyful tears. TEARS OF HOPE!! There was a smile on her face. She believed and desired hope for me. I could feel it in my soul, as tears were running down my face. I didn't expect her singing. I wasn't sure what to expect. One of the best presentations Debra displayed was coming from the place of love that she possessed for me. I was beginning to feel the power of the shower. My heart was filled with hope. Before they were just words, now I am starting to feel where I want to be. I began to have a sense of something to live for. As we finished the song, everyone else began to sing the words as the tears of joy and hope to come across in their eyes. From siting inside this circle I was receiving nothing but good energy.

Pastor Fuller concluded the shower with words of encouragement for me and my family. The roles that everyone would play in this process were very clear. Chores had been assigned to reliable attendees, which was a load off of my shoulders. And, I had already felt liberated – as though the cancer was out of my body: simply by knowing that I would be supported from my friends and family – a thing that is shared in this technologically-advanced world through text, Social Media or emails. My mom and Aunt Elizabeth are extremely spiritual ladies, and they affirmed that God will always rise to the occasion. Both agreed that I was going to be blessed with perfect health. They affirmed that I would live a life as long as their lives. This cancer was just part of the journey of life – something to help me grow: to help me reach a higher place of knowing and understanding my faith and belief in God.

My shower ended with a pot luck-style banquet, and it was fabulous. I think that the rays of energy made my appetite increase. Much-needed dialogue took place. While eating, folks shared their pleasing experiences from the shower. Many wanted to help, and felt this shower offered the best structure for assisting others during times of need. Cancer was no longer this taboo subject that we couldn't mention. We talked about it, and now we know how to deal with it together as one!

> *Everything that is done in the world is done by hope.*
> *-* **Martin Luther**

The Healing Shower

Letters from Family Members
Rickey (Husband)

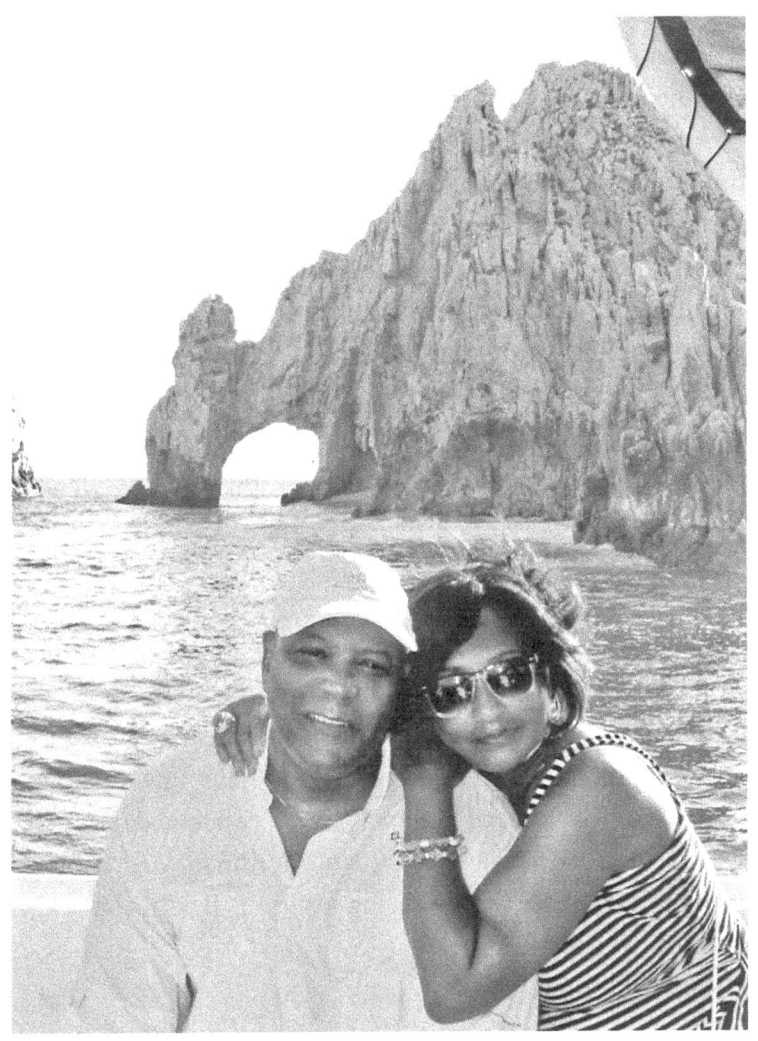

Eloise Laws

To My Dearest El:

There are two attributes I have always loved about you; undaunted optimism and ability to always look on the bright side of life. Not that you aren't an emotional person, but I believe the reason I have seldom seen you cry in the 30-plus years that we have been together is because of these attributes. You can understand then how my heart sank, when after you told me about your diagnosis: you laid your head on my shoulder and cried.

I felt helpless, powerless and deep sadness – like the kind that only comes from a broken heart. As I stood there holding you close to me, I felt my spirit not only fill with despair but also fear. What next? Could I lose you? Where do we go from here? How do I support you in the face of this critical and frightening reality? We embraced and held each other motionless, oblivious to time. Then, at some point you stopped crying. You slowly raised your head, looked into my eyes and said, "No, we're going to get through this." Your words seemed to lift both of our spirits. I felt relief. Your optimism would not let you stay down too long. I smiled faintly, and responded, "Yes, we will."

We had some tough times ahead of us but, we got through them. But in those first few timeless moments, after learning about your condition, I felt every emotion. I would experience through the entire ordeal; despair, sadness, heartache, fear, resolve and the realization that the only thing I could do to help you was to embrace you and love you. Along the way, you conceived your ***Healing Shower*** concept as a way to build up optimism and a bright side perspective for anyone who is facing a serious health challenge. I am so proud of you for turning your own misfortune into a beacon of confidence and brightness for others.

God Bless You El,
Your Loving Husband,
With All My Love,
For All My Life

The Healing Shower

Mother (Miola)

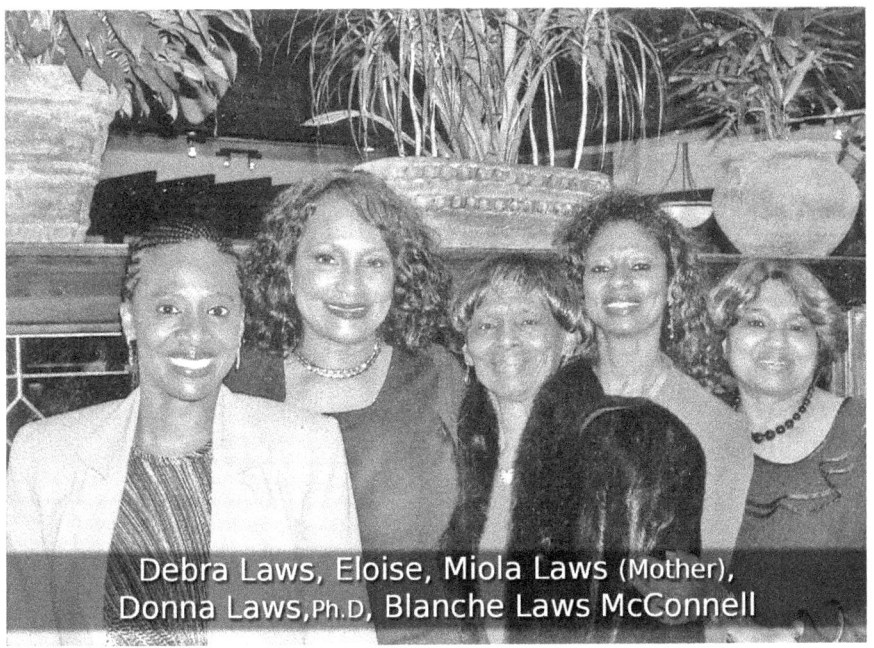

Debra Laws, Eloise, Miola Laws (Mother), Donna Laws, Ph.D, Blanche Laws McConnell

To My Lovely, Courageous Daughter Eloise:

We still manage to remain a very, close-knit family. In spite of the geographical distance you and the other siblings on the West Coast are, and I remaining in Texas. Through frequent visits and various technical communication methods, we constantly stay in touch.

As my motherly vibes kick in, I've always, by the sound of your voice in your phone calls, could sense what was going on in your life. Your sisters and brothers skillfully tried to keep you away from me, and when they decided that they could not keep your secret any longer, I got the phone call.

Eloise, you know you all were taught that prayer, faith and GOD's power would and could help us through all difficulties. Sometimes, a person does not know what they are made of, or what they can stand until it happens. Life can be altered from what you even expected it to be. You may have known others who experienced receiving such life-altering news: but not in a million years imagined it could be happening to you. This whole ordeal seems like we just saw a horror movie: but this was for real. You are the real character of the movie. This is your life, and you had to fight to keep it.

Eloise, it caused me to seek GOD like never before! I had to push the replay button of my mind's recordings and play back all the times GOD has brought this family through difficult times. And recall the many victories He has given us over problems that seemed impossible to solve. Death was not an option. WE would get through this cancer victoriously! I knew GOD would not fail us: prayer and faith always works! WE would fight and win the battle. We fought and won. Thanks be to GOD for our victory! You are a very strong Christian woman.

GOD Bless!
Love,
Mother

The Healing Shower

Alexx Ivie (Daughter)

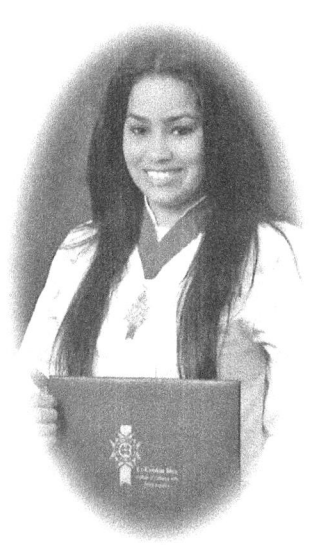

I felt upset that my mom kept this from me for so long. I now understand why she did it. I was afraid for my mom and didn't think there was anything I could do except pray. I isolated myself many times due to me being frightened about the outcome of her diagnosis, and subsequent result: but, harbored massive amounts of confusion. As a result, my introspective reaction caused my family to turn against me. During my isolated times, I prayed and prayed which I believed helped! Now, mom has a perfect boob. A perfect melon — no cancer.

And, I pray it is gone forever (ETERNALLY ERADICATED). I can help her through this by giving love, and the little things I can do that she is incapable of doing for herself ... such as: removing her slippers when she relaxes and prepares for bed, removing her lunch or dinner tray so she won't have to struggle to get up and down out of her favorite chair, you know, little detailed things that adults find hard to do. Or, just don't want to do if there is a kid around. My mom will definitely try to take advantage of that. That's why you have to love her. And, I do.

Eloise Laws

Donna "Dr. D" (Younger Sister)

Dear Eloise,

From a little girl, I always admired your beauty and your style. I looked up to you from afar, knowing you were my sister. But also, as someone I didn't really know, but always excited to see! I vividly remember one night, as I lay in bed and began to suck my thumb. Mother lay beside me and said, "If you continue to suck your thumb, you will not grow up to look pretty like Eloise." I thought to myself, "Oh, no!" So, I asked Mother to watch me that night as I slept, to make sure I would not suck my thumb. I felt in my sleep throughout the night, pulling my thumb away from my mouth. As Mother and Dad tried tirelessly, everything they knew to make me stop sucking my thumb. If they had only known, all it took was those few words.

From that night on, my thumb-sucking ceased. At that time, I discovered the strength and willpower I had, and how one's belief can get one through anything. That same strong belief in GOD and my Faith is what took me through this journey with you.

The day you told me you had to go back to the doctor to have a breast biopsy after you had your mammogram, I immediately thought and felt, "This is not good." But, in doing what I always choose to do with life and its challenges, I erred on the side of optimism and my Faith in GOD. I first prayed that GOD would keep you, heal you, and bring you through whatever this test would be. I then made certain that my calendar was clear to be with you the entire day of your biopsy.

As I go back to timely recollect the events that were to befall us, it all seems to be a blur, with the exception of specific moments. As we waited in anticipation for the results, the day you called me and said you got the phone call from the doctor, I already knew when I heard the silence in the sound of your voice as you tried to be courageous in your words.

The Healing Shower

The results came back positive for breast cancer – Ductal Carcinoma Insitu (DCIS). At that time, I came over - for I just wanted to be by your side. As I sat at the bar, while you were right across in the kitchen, I was saddened and felt a deep lowness in my heart. But, for some reason, I did not fret. My thoughts then went to a moment that I remembered years ago. Mother told me, that a premonition came to her that a daughter, (you Eloise), would have cancer.

As you know, we all go to Mother as our confidant (our brothers included), because her intuitions run deep and true. Some things we want to hear, and some we don't. Nevertheless, she is a strong woman of GOD with tremendous Faith. And, GOD does not steer her wrong. I have to say, I am Blessed in that GOD has chosen to use me in the same way. So, with that, I kicked into survival mode, for I knew that was just what you were going to be… A Survivor! I said to you, "I know I'm your baby sister, but I got this!" I notified our other sisters and brothers, feeling her pain and sorrow, and asked that they not reveal this to Mother. However, that would not last for long. Within a couple of days, her motherly intuition kicked in. She called me and specifically asked me if everything was okay, and if something was wrong with you (Eloise).

Once, I got past telling her what she already knew, I put on my medical/health hat. I thank GOD for the medical experience, understanding, and knowledge He has given me, so that I could be liaison and voice between you and your medical doctors, for your medical care. I consider it to be a Blessing to be there every step of the way to effectively communicate between the doctors and family. I was determined to seek out the best doctors and care from M.D. Anderson Cancer Center in Houston, Texas, to UCLA Medical Center in Los Angeles, Calif. I began my research, gathering information, and making phone calls to figure out just what was this DCIS. And yes, as I scheduled appointments for you, you cancelled them. Knowing that you were simply facing the common stages of questioning and denial, I stayed steadfast in my quest. Yes, baby sister stepped into big sister's shoes. You soon reached the stages of acceptance, and the journey continued from there. After much homework, doctor consults, and thought, it was decided for you to have a double mastectomy to ensure a lesser prognosis of recurrence, and a higher level of survival.

Prior to the surgery, you came up with a most creative idea of having, the **Healing Shower**. It was to be a time when family, friends and loved ones bring you well-wishes, and inspirational gestures before undergoing surgery, medical procedures, or at times of severe illnesses, and on into the recuperative period. Your **Healing Shower** was the most uplifting and inspirational gathering of love, family, and friends.

Well, it was that time. Early on Tuesday morning, Nov. 13, 2007, Mother, Debra, and I were there to pick you up and drive you to the hospital. As you were standing in the garage waiting, I remember seeing you as a brave soldier ready for a battle that you knew you had already won. You remained steadfast from the time they rolled you in for pre-operation preparation, up to the surgery. At that moment, before taking you in, you expressed to me that you changed your mind. You did not want a double mastectomy. I encouraged you to do what you strongly desired, and that the final decision was yours. After much prayer, the support of your family and friends, and many hours of waiting, you came through as the shining star you are. The first thing you said was, "I'm so glad I didn't let them take both of my breasts."

As you went through the days of recovery and follow-ups, I knew there were times of the unknown, reflection, and still unanswered questions. But, you remained upbeat and at peace. And, let us not forget your strength and belief in the Almighty power of GOD. He who has made you the woman of GOD that you are has allowed you to tell your story time and time again through word, talent, and deed, and be a testimony to others. It is all for His Glory.

When Praises go up, Blessings come down. I smile with gratitude when I can say, my sister is a Survivor!

The Healing Shower

Continue to let our FATHER use you my sister … Strong Woman of GOD.

I love you sis!
Your "baby" sis,
Donna "Dr. D"

Blanche (Older Sister)

My Dearest Sister Eloise,

    Upon learning of your diagnosis, my first reaction (and I'm sure the family's reaction) was, "Why Eloise? Why us?" However, I was quickly reminded of a former co-worker of mine, who when he was diagnosed, his response was, "Why not me?" I also reminded myself that Eloise has cancer: Cancer does not have her.

    Thank GOD, Eloise for your idea of a ***Healing Shower.*** I know that not only were you blessed with ever-increasing faith, so were we.

    We all go through times of sadness, sorrow and tears. GOD draws close to us in tenderness during those times. GOD does not want us to live a tear-filled life. Tears are for the night, but joy comes in the morning.

    It is no accident that you survived. Today, you are in GOD's place, in GOD's time, to fulfill GOD's plan, in GOD's way, by GOD's grace, for GOD's glory. You are the Lord's.

    Healing is a blessing from GOD and so is good health. In so many ways, GOD expresses His grace and mercies to you, touching you in your need and time again. He renews your strength, restores your well-being, revives your heart, refreshes your spirit, and relaxes your nerves. So, keep singing, keep smiling, knowing you can always count on GOD, for sure.

Lots of Love and Prayers Always,
Your Big Sister,
Blanche

The Healing Shower

Debra (Younger Sister)

Dear Eloise,

    Some memories of the past are just too painful to bring forward. All the work you do to put them away seems like a lifetime of therapy only to have to recall the unthinkable. Every time I sit down to write, I find myself getting up to do other things: making excuses not to. So, here's to the best of my recollection when I got the news of your breast cancer diagnosis….

    I literally fell to my knees, screaming and praying to GOD to not let it be true! I thought I stopped breathing because I felt numb. You see, this was only the reaction to the preliminary diagnosis. A biopsy would be needed to confirm the preliminary results. Just a few weeks prior to this, I had a scary episode of my own regarding a test I needed to take (CEA) blood test. I let my imagination get the best of me and before I knew it, I had pronounced my own death sentence. I was so relieved to get a negative result, and NOW THIS!!

    I was visiting Mother at home in Houston, Texas, at the time. We were at the grocery store when my cell phone rang. Eloise was on the other end with broken words in her voice, as she stated that she had just left the doctor's office. It was confirmed that she has breast cancer…

    I was pushing the grocery cart and Mother was close by. I could not let her see or hear my reaction. It was all I could or could not do to let go. Moments of silence followed by … somehow, I had to gather myself. I told her I would call her back. It's very difficult to hide anything from Mother, as she swears her strong intuitions in the form of premonitions are always on target. Later, I would learn from Mother when she said, "I already knew it was breast cancer," before I had to tell her, being in such a fragile state of health.

    Mother said she had a dream some years earlier that one of her daughters would have cancer! We didn't know what kind: later to find out it was breast cancer. You see, this disease does not run in my family. I wanted so desperately to pack up and get back to L.A., but Mother was recovering from knee replacement surgery. You know what they say, "When it rains, it pours!" Everything's in total chaos! I guess GOD put me exactly where I needed to be at the time.

Meanwhile, my other two sisters were in L.A. with Eloise. As soon as Mother was able to travel, we left for L.A. Mother was a strong woman, in faith and otherwise. She was always putting the interest of others before herself. Being the prayer warrior that she is, she had to get to her daughter!! Now, the real test came to show what this family is made of - especially the sisters. We do what we always do – we united in prayer. Mother took control, giving us strength that she receives from our Heavenly Father. Only He can give us the power beyond what is normal of what we can bear to be able to endure.

When we arrived in L.A., my youngest sister Donna had done all the preliminary work of setting up doctors' appointments for various tests to be performed, gathering all the necessary information to make the best informed decisions for treatments. When you have a patient that has been diagnosed, you literally have to take over and think for them, while she is trying to keep her eyes open and dry. It is an overwhelming feeling we have to shoulder up for them.

From consultations with the doctors, we all agree, the best plan of action is to have a double-mastectomy. Although she was only in Stage 1, she didn't want to do a repeat performance of another surgery later, and because of the DCIS (Ductal Carcinoma In-Situ) we wanted to be sure we got it all. The night before the surgery, the family put together with friends an event, "Celebration," later to be called ***The Healing Shower***. It's a celebration of well-wishes from friends and family, where everyone expresses in whatever form they choose, to uplift Eloise (and other patients).

Heartfelt sentiments and prayers were expressed, along with song and praise – and this was all filmed! The love that filled that room was most inspirational, which put Eloise in a position to receive her blessings to come!! I chose to sing a song I felt was most

The Healing Shower

fitting for this occasion called, "I Hope You Dance." She loved it! (smile)

The morning of the scheduled surgery, we leave early for the hospital with Eloise. Dear friends come from all over to support a brave little soldier! We are all at the waiting room area as we observe others, waiting for their loved ones to come out or go into surgery. We say a prayer before Eloise goes into the prep room, and send hugs and kisses to her. Now, at the last minute before she is to be wheeled into the operating room, Eloise decides she only wants one (1) breast removed! OK it's her prerogative!!! The rest is embracing the journey of survival that lies ahead together in unity my sweet sister!

With all my heart I salute you Eloise!
May God continue to bless and fortify you! (smile)
Debra

Awards & Recognition

Eloise Laws

Eloise Laws

S T A T E O F C A L I F O R N I A

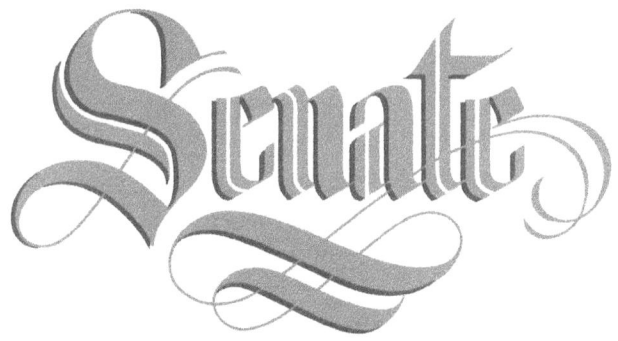

CERTIFICATE OF RECOGNITION

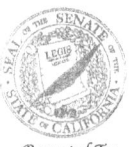

Presented To:

Eloise Laws

****

On the occasion of being honored by the

Harry A. Mier AbilityFirst Center

*and in recognition of your outstanding leadership
and exemplary service throughout our community
Congratulations and best wishes for continued success!*

"A Musical Extravaganza"
July 15, 2012
Inglewood, California

RODERICK D. WRIGHT
MEMBER OF THE SENATE, 25TH DISTRICT
CALIFORNIA STATE LEGISLATURE

*State Senate Certificate of Recognition Awarded to
Eloise Laws, July 15, 2012*

The Healing Shower

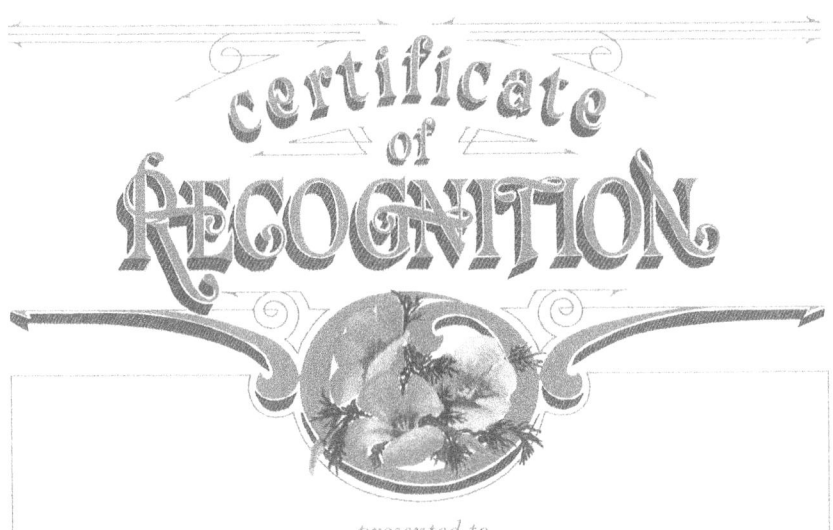

CALIFORNIA STATE SENATE

Certificate of Recognition

presented to

Eloise Laws

*World Renowned
Award-Winning Vocalist*

On behalf of myself and the constituents of the 26th Senate District, I would like to commend you for your support and work on behalf of The AbilityFirst Harry A. Mier Center and for all you do to serve the needs of children and adults with disabilities in our community. Wishing you continued success in all your future endeavors.

Dated this 15th Day of July 2012
Senator Curren D. Price Jr.
26th Senate District

Senator

*California State Senate - Eloise Laws
World Renowned Award-Winning Vocalist, July 15, 2012*

Eloise Laws

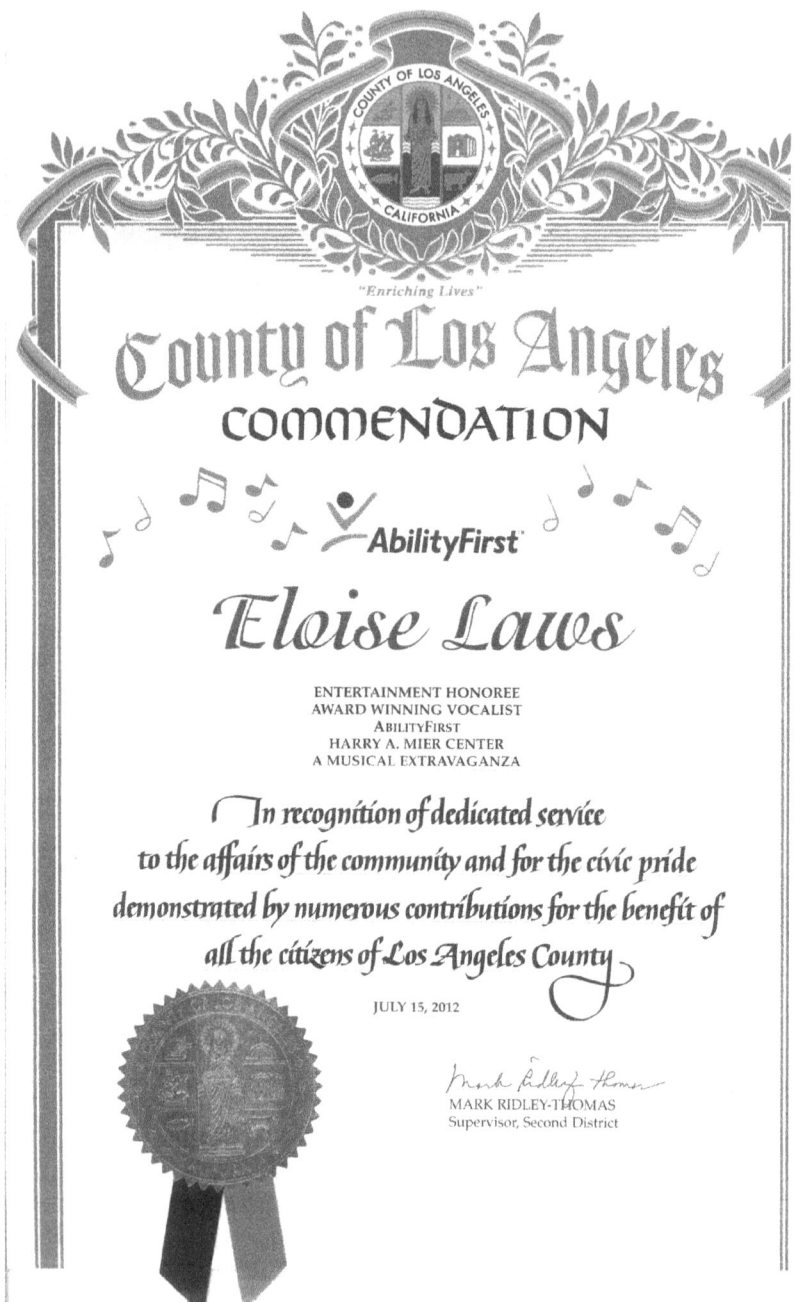

County of Los Angeles Commendation Awarded to Eloise Laws - July 15, 2012

The Healing Shower

Congratulations

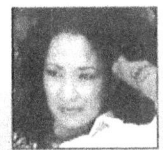

Eloise Laws Ivie
on receiving the
SYREETA WRIGHT-MUHAMMAD
PIONEER FOR THE CURE AWARD

and to

THE DENISE ROBERTS
BREAST CANCER FOUNDATION

for 10 years of service as advocates to
the cause, the care and the cure

IMW
IVIE, MCNEILL & WYATT

Rickey Ivie Robert H. McNeill, Jr. W. Keith Wyatt
Eulanda L. Matthews Byron M. Purcell
Rupert A. Byrdsong

Allison Turner Ben Davis Davida Frieman
Diana Taing Jennifer Jacobs Lilia Duchrow
Peter Carr IV Randy Kennon Teresa Hillery
Venus Trunnel Wendy Wu

Eloise received the Syreeta Wright - Muhammad Award - Pioneer for the Cure Award

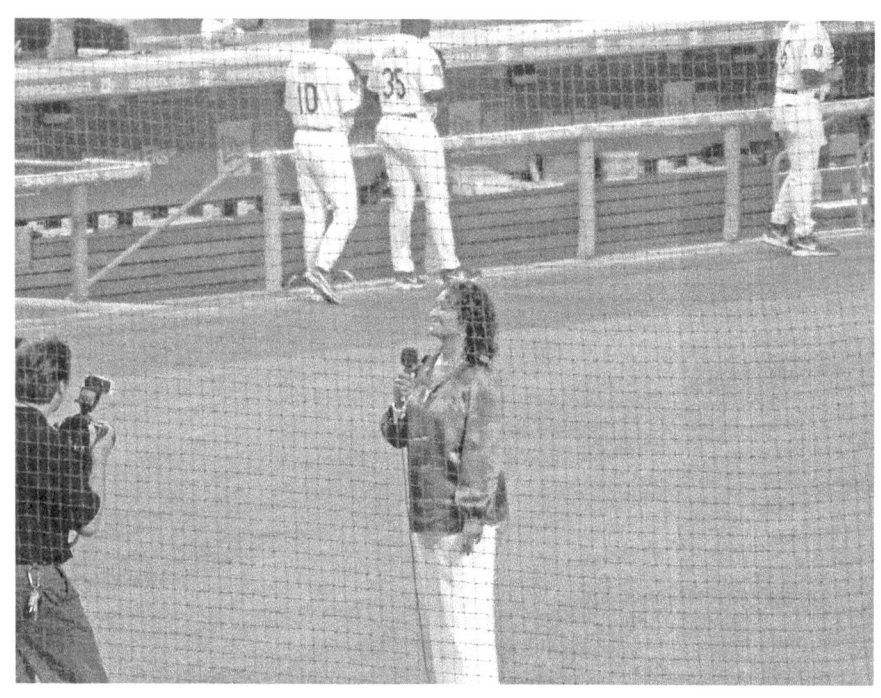

Eloise performing at the Los Angeles Dodger Stadium in 2009

The Healing Shower

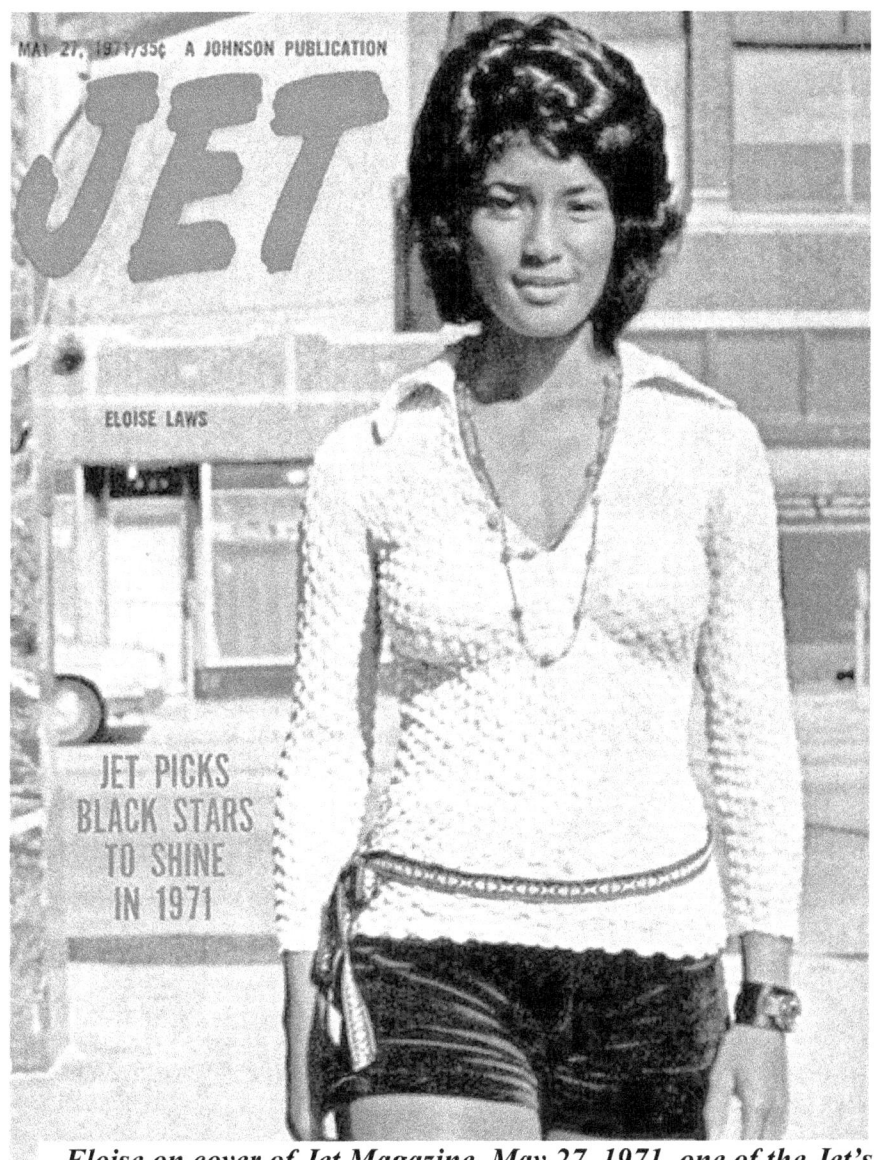

Eloise on cover of Jet Magazine, May 27, 1971, one of the Jet's Picks of Black Stars to Shine in 1971

Getting Your House in Order

Will/Living Trust

It is imperative to have these documents prepared in advance if at all possible. You'll find examples at the end of the book.

Power of Attorney/Advance Health Care Directive

Before entering the hospital to receive treatment for any serious condition or surgery pertaining to cancer, heart disease or transplant, it is necessary to have all legal documents pertaining to Beneficiaries or and/or Advance Health Care Directive properly secured, where a designated person can find them. I have seen many Family Feuds because loved ones don't know the difference between these two documents. An Advance Health Care Directive does not have the same "power" or position as the person who has Power of Attorney. At the same time, you can reverse Power of Attorney, if you get permission or documents to do so. You'll find examples of both documents at the end of the book.

Be sure to prepare your documents correctly to prevent any and all feuding between all of your family members. **Please remind your relatives to refrain from carrying any weapons or sharp objects to the funeral and/or gravesite!

RECOVERY SECTION

Managing Side Effects

These are some of the side effects that are common to chemotherapy and some tips for managing them:
- Dry skin and rashes
- Mouth sores
- Hot flashes
- Sexuality
- Depression
- Hair loss if radiation treatment is involved.
- Dealing with hair loss.
    - Get short hair cuts
    - Shop for wigs
    - Be gentle with your hair using mild but the best shampoos and soft hair brushes.
    - Avoid chemicals if radiation is involved.
    - Shaving your head before your hair loss or before it starts to fall out.

Remember you have and can wear an array of beautiful scarves and hats or turbans. You may decide to not cover at all.

Gastrointestinal side-effects:

A. Decreased appetite

B. Diarrhea

C. Constipation

D. Anxiety

E. Pain

F. Peripheral neuropathy. Certain drugs may affect the nerves in your body — hands, knees, feet, burning sensations. It's very important to report these symptoms to your health care team.

THE SEVEN LEVELS OF HEALING

1. Education and Information

2. Connection with others

3. The Body as a Garden (Nutrition on a daily basis)

4. Emotional Healing

5. **Nature {OR NUTURE/FROM JAZZ BOOK}** of the Body and Mind

6. Life assessment

7. Nurture the spirit

About the Author

Eloise Laws is an incomparable, world-renowned, award-winning vocalist, Tony-nominated actress, author, and breast cancer survivor. For more than 30 years, this angelic, versatile performer has been gracing stages such as; the Playboy Jazz Festival; Tokyo, Japan's famed Cotton Club; 94.7FM's Jazz By the Bay on the Queen Mary; Tom Joyner's Fantastic Voyage Cruise (2007); *Royal Caribbean's* "Freedom of the Seas"; and the Atlanta Jazz Festival. Highly-requested at music festivals, Laws is also a winner of the prestigious Cherry Blossom Award from the Tokyo Music Festival. A dynamic vocalist, her unique style and expression is an infusion of blues, jazz, R&B, soul, rock, and reggae, which harmoniously floats between paradise and serenity.

Produced by such luminaries as Holland-Dozier-Holland, Linda Creed, Andre Fisher, and Ronnie Laws, Laws can be heard on several classic Capital, Liberty and ABC recordings. As co-writer and original lead actress (Gretha Boston) of the 1999, Tony-nominated musical, *It Ain't Nothin' But the Blues*, Laws helped garner four Tony nominations. Among the Tony nominations, her lead role as Gretha earned a Tony nod for Best Performance by a Featured Actress in a Musical. Laws also received a coveted nomination for a Drama Desk Award in the category of Outstanding Featured Actress in a Musical, as well as a nomination for the Helen Hayes Award for Best Actress in Outstanding Non-Resident Production.

Eloise Laws

In this debut book, **The Healing Shower**, Laws shares her personal journey, surviving the "ups and downs" of breast cancer. Inspired by the outpouring of love and support she received from family and friends, prompted Laws to write this heart-felt account. Included are all of the tools one who is suffering from a life-threatening illness will need as a guide. From developing an Action Team, where you cultivate a group to help make life-changing decisions; to creating a Good Deeds and Services/Sign-up List for loved ones to assist you before and after surgery (i.e. grocery shopping, feeding your pets, cooking meals); **The Healing Shower** is a teaching manual offering much-needed advice about how loved ones and friends can offer their services and be held accountable during a crucial time. Hopefully, readers will have a better understanding about how they can assist those recovering from cancer.

Laws is married to Attorney Rickey Ivie, and they have a daughter, Alexx. The family lives in Southern California.

www.eloiselaws.com

Recommended Classes / Support Groups

Mind/Body/Spirit/Workshops

Drumming Circles, www.remo.com
661-294-5600 – Remo, Inc., an industry leader in percussion instruments, also offers research in healing through drumming. Visit the website or call for Breast Cancer Drumming Circles in your area.

Hynoptherapy/Tapping
Learn the basics of self-hypnosis and Emotional Therapy Freedom Technique (EFT). Tapping on certain parts of the body helps to let go of negative energy.

Tai Chi or (Tai Chi Chuan), http://www.chenbing.org,
1144 S. Western Ave., Los Angeles, Ca 90006 – Also known as Taijiquan is a slow-moving form of martial arts with a healing component known to help breast cancer survivors live healthier lives. The Chen Bing Taiji Academy is a leading martial arts academy in the discipline of Tai Chi taught by Master Chen Bing, who is a direct descent of Taijiquan creator Chen Wangting.

YOGA
No two classes are alike, however, this is truly a healing experience. Speak with your doctor about the best type of yoga that's conducive to your recovery. Some practitioners will even make home visits. Namaste.

Eloise Laws

Support Groups

Susan G. Komen,
http://ww5.komen.org/BreastCancer/SupportGroups.html
The Susan G. Komen page is comprehensive in its offerings from treatment advice; to support groups; to insurance and financial issues.

Breast Cancer Organization,
http://www.breastcancer.org/questions/support
Centralized site offers information on how to find local breast cancer support groups.
https://www.herceptin.com/breast/resources
Offers online support from registered oncology nurses 24/7 to patients receiving Herceptin treatment for Breast Cancer.

Army of Women Research Foundation,
http://www.dslrf.org/army/
Dr. Susan Love Research Foundation offers an innovative approach to ending the cure by conducting more than 20 studies, as well as educating the public and advocacy. 310-828-0060 (local) or 1-866-569-0388.

The Denise Roberts Foundation
http://tdrbcf.org
888-8- DENISE (1-888-833-6473) - The Denise Roberts Breast Cancer Foundation (TDRBCF) is a 501 (c) – (3) nonprofit organization, which exists to change the mindfulness of women and men of color, to one of health and self-awareness. Being breast cancer-free for more than 20 years, Denise Roberts strives to ensure cancer patients are aware of their choices, and assists in helping them make wise lifestyle decisions.

Women of Color, Breast Cancer Organization of Inglewood, Calif.,
301 N. Prarie Ave., Inglewood, Calif., 90301.

Annual Calendar
Appointments, Classes, Events and Notes

January Week 1

Faith - Psalm 143 - NLT - A psalm of David. - Hear my prayer, O LORD; listen to my plea! Answer me because you are faithful and righteous.

SUNDAY	
MONDAY	
TUESDAY	
WEDNESDAY	
THURSDAY	
FRIDAY	
SATURDAY	

Eloise Laws

January Week 2

Faith - Psalm 143 - NLT - A psalm of David. - Hear my prayer, O LORD; listen to my plea! Answer me because you are faithful and righteous.

SUNDAY	
MONDAY	
TUESDAY	
WEDNESDAY	
THURSDAY	
FRIDAY	
SATURDAY	

The Healing Shower

January Week 3

Faith - Psalm 143 - NLT - A psalm of David. - Hear my prayer, O LORD; listen to my plea! Answer me because you are faithful and righteous.

SUNDAY	
MONDAY	
TUESDAY	
WEDNESDAY	
THURSDAY	
FRIDAY	
SATURDAY	

Eloise Laws

January Week 4

Faith - Psalm 143 - NL - A psalm of David. - Hear my prayer, O LORD; listen to my plea! Answer me because you are faithful and righteous.

SUNDAY	
MONDAY	
TUESDAY	
WEDNESDAY	
THURSDAY	
FRIDAY	
SATURDAY	

The Healing Shower

February Week 1

Trust - Passage 2 Samuel 22:3 - NLT - ... ... my God is my rock, in whom I find protection. He is my shield, the power that saves me, and my place of safety. He is my refuge, my savior, the one who saves me from violence.

SUNDAY	
MONDAY	
TUESDAY	
WEDNESDAY	
THURSDAY	
FRIDAY	
SATURDAY	

Eloise Laws

February Week 2

Trust - Passage 2 Samuel 22:3 - NLT - ... ... my God is my rock, in whom I find protection. He is my shield, the power that saves me, and my place of safety. He is my refuge, my savior, the one who saves me from violence.

SUNDAY	
MONDAY	
TUESDAY	
WEDNESDAY	
THURSDAY	
FRIDAY	
SATURDAY	

The Healing Shower

February Week 3

Trust - Passage 2 Samuel 22:3 - NLT - ... ... my God is my rock, in whom I find protection. He is my shield, the power that saves me, and my place of safety. He is my refuge, my savior, the one who saves me from violence.

SUNDAY	
MONDAY	
TUESDAY	
WEDNESDAY	
THURSDAY	
FRIDAY	
SATURDAY	

February Week 4

Trust - Passage 2 Samuel 22:3 - NLT - ... ... my God is my rock, in whom I find protection. He is my shield, the power that saves me, and my place of safety. He is my refuge, my savior, the one who saves me from violence.

SUNDAY

MONDAY

TUESDAY

WEDNESDAY

THURSDAY

FRIDAY

SATURDAY

The Healing Shower

March Week 1

Peace - Passage Judges 6:23 - Amp. - The Lord said to him, Peace be to you, do not fear; you shall not die.

SUNDAY	
MONDAY	
TUESDAY	
WEDNESDAY	
THURSDAY	
FRIDAY	
SATURDAY	

March Week 2

Peace - Passage Judges 6:23 - Amp. - The Lord said to him, Peace be to you, do not fear; you shall not die.

SUNDAY	
MONDAY	
TUESDAY	
WEDNESDAY	
THURSDAY	
FRIDAY	
SATURDAY	

The Healing Shower

March Week 3

Peace - Passage Judges 6:23 - Amp. - The Lord said to him, Peace be to you, do not fear; you shall not die.

SUNDAY	
MONDAY	
TUESDAY	
WEDNESDAY	
THURSDAY	
FRIDAY	
SATURDAY	

March Week 4

Peace - Passage Judges 6:23 - Amp. - The Lord said to him, Peace be to you, do not fear; you shall not die.

SUNDAY	
MONDAY	
TUESDAY	
WEDNESDAY	
THURSDAY	
FRIDAY	
SATURDAY	

The Healing Shower

April Week 1

Hope - Psalm 119:116 - NLT - LORD, sustain me as you promised, that I may live! Do not let my hope be crushed.

SUNDAY	
MONDAY	
TUESDAY	
WEDNESDAY	
THURSDAY	
FRIDAY	
SATURDAY	

Eloise Laws

April Week 2

Hope - Psalm 119:116 - NL - LORD, sustain me as you promised, that I may live! Do not let my hope be crushed.

SUNDAY	
MONDAY	
TUESDAY	
WEDNESDAY	
THURSDAY	
FRIDAY	
SATURDAY	

The Healing Shower

April Week 3

Hope - Psalm 119:116 - NLT - LORD, sustain me as you promised, that I may live! Do not let my hope be crushed.

SUNDAY	
MONDAY	
TUESDAY	
WEDNESDAY	
THURSDAY	
FRIDAY	
SATURDAY	

Eloise Laws

April Week 4

Hope - Psalm 119:116 - NLT - LORD, sustain me as you promised, that I may live! Do not let my hope be crushed.

SUNDAY	
MONDAY	
TUESDAY	
WEDNESDAY	
THURSDAY	
FRIDAY	
SATURDAY	

The Healing Shower

May Week 1

Endurance - Colossians 1:11 - Amp. - [We pray] that you may be invigorated and strengthened with all power according to the might of His glory, [to exercise] every kind of endurance and patience (perseverance and forbearance) with joy,

SUNDAY	
MONDAY	
TUESDAY	
WEDNESDAY	
THURSDAY	
FRIDAY	
SATURDAY	

Eloise Laws

May Week 2

Endurance - Colossians 1:11 - Amp. - [We pray] that you may be invigorated and strengthened with all power according to the might of His glory, [to exercise] every kind of endurance and patience (perseverance and forbearance) with joy,

SUNDAY	
MONDAY	
TUESDAY	
WEDNESDAY	
THURSDAY	
FRIDAY	
SATURDAY	

The Healing Shower

May Week 3

Endurance - Colossians 1:11 - Amp. - [We pray] that you may be invigorated and strengthened with all power according to the might of His glory, [to exercise] every kind of endurance and patience (perseverance and forbearance) with joy,

SUNDAY	
MONDAY	
TUESDAY	
WEDNESDAY	
THURSDAY	
FRIDAY	
SATURDAY	

Eloise Laws

May Week 4

Endurance - Colossians 1:11 - Amp. - [We pray] that you may be invigorated and strengthened with all power according to the might of His glory, [to exercise] every kind of endurance and patience (perseverance and forbearance) with joy,

SUNDAY	
MONDAY	
TUESDAY	
WEDNESDAY	
THURSDAY	
FRIDAY	
SATURDAY	

June Week 1

Joy - Habakkuk 3:18 - NLT - ... yet I will rejoice in the LORD! I will be joyful in the God of my salvation!

SUNDAY	
MONDAY	
TUESDAY	
WEDNESDAY	
THURSDAY	
FRIDAY	
SATURDAY	

June Week 2

Joy - Habakkuk 3:18 - NLT - ... yet I will rejoice in the LORD!
I will be joyful in the God of my salvation!

SUNDAY	
MONDAY	
TUESDAY	
WEDNESDAY	
THURSDAY	
FRIDAY	
SATURDAY	

The Healing Shower

June Week 3

Joy - Habakkuk 3:18 - NLT - ... yet I will rejoice in the LORD!
I will be joyful in the God of my salvation!

SUNDAY	
MONDAY	
TUESDAY	
WEDNESDAY	
THURSDAY	
FRIDAY	
SATURDAY	

Eloise Laws

June Week 4

Joy - Habakkuk 3:18 - NL - ... yet I will rejoice in the LORD! I will be joyful in the God of my salvation!

SUNDAY	
MONDAY	
TUESDAY	
WEDNESDAY	
THURSDAY	
FRIDAY	
SATURDAY	

The Healing Shower

July Week 1

Grateful - Acts 24:3 - NLT - For all of this, Your Excellency, we are very grateful to you.

SUNDAY	
MONDAY	
TUESDAY	
WEDNESDAY	
THURSDAY	
FRIDAY	
SATURDAY	

July Week 2

Grateful - Acts 24:3 - NL - For all of this, Your Excellency, we are very grateful to you.

SUNDAY	
MONDAY	
TUESDAY	
WEDNESDAY	
THURSDAY	
FRIDAY	
SATURDAY	

The Healing Shower

July Week 3

Grateful - Acts 24:3 - NL - For all of this, Your Excellency, we are very grateful to you.

SUNDAY	
MONDAY	
TUESDAY	
WEDNESDAY	
THURSDAY	
FRIDAY	
SATURDAY	

Eloise Laws

July Week 4

Grateful - Acts 24:3 - NL - For all of this, Your Excellency, we are very grateful to you.

SUNDAY	
MONDAY	
TUESDAY	
WEDNESDAY	
THURSDAY	
FRIDAY	
SATURDAY	

The Healing Shower

August Week 1

Mercy - Psalm 28:2 - NLT - Listen to my prayer for mercy as I cry out to you for help, as I lift my hands toward your holy sanctuary.

SUNDAY	
MONDAY	
TUESDAY	
WEDNESDAY	
THURSDAY	
FRIDAY	
SATURDAY	

August Week 2

Mercy - Psalm 28:2 - NLT - Listen to my prayer for mercy as I cry out to you for help, as I lift my hands toward your holy sanctuary.

SUNDAY	
MONDAY	
TUESDAY	
WEDNESDAY	
THURSDAY	
FRIDAY	
SATURDAY	

The Healing Shower

August Week 3

Mercy - Psalm 28:2 - NLT - Listen to my prayer for mercy as I cry out to you for help, as I lift my hands toward your holy sanctuary.

SUNDAY	
MONDAY	
TUESDAY	
WEDNESDAY	
THURSDAY	
FRIDAY	
SATURDAY	

August Week 4

Mercy - Psalm 28:2 - NLT - Listen to my prayer for mercy as I cry out to you for help, as I lift my hands toward your holy sanctuary.

SUNDAY	
MONDAY	
TUESDAY	
WEDNESDAY	
THURSDAY	
FRIDAY	
SATURDAY	

The Healing Shower

September Week 1

Grace - Acts 20:24 - NLT - But my life is worth nothing to me unless I use it for finishing the work assigned me by the Lord Jesus—the work of telling others the Good News about the wonderful grace of God.

SUNDAY	
MONDAY	
TUESDAY	
WEDNESDAY	
THURSDAY	
FRIDAY	
SATURDAY	

Eloise Laws

September Week 2

Grace - Acts 20:24 - NLT - But my life is worth nothing to me unless I use it for finishing the work assigned me by the Lord Jesus—the work of telling others the Good News about the wonderful grace of God.

SUNDAY	
MONDAY	
TUESDAY	
WEDNESDAY	
THURSDAY	
FRIDAY	
SATURDAY	

The Healing Shower

September Week 3

Grace - Acts 20:24 - NLT - But my life is worth nothing to me unless I use it for finishing the work assigned me by the Lord Jesus—the work of telling others the Good News about the wonderful grace of God.

SUNDAY	
MONDAY	
TUESDAY	
WEDNESDAY	
THURSDAY	
FRIDAY	
SATURDAY	

Eloise Laws

September Week 4

Grace - Acts 20:24 - NLT - But my life is worth nothing to me unless I use it for finishing the work assigned me by the Lord Jesus—the work of telling others the Good News about the wonderful grace of God.

SUNDAY	
MONDAY	
TUESDAY	
WEDNESDAY	
THURSDAY	
FRIDAY	
SATURDAY	

The Healing Shower

October Week 1

Patience - Ecclesiastes 7:8 - NLT - Finishing is better than starting. Patience is better than pride.

SUNDAY	
MONDAY	
TUESDAY	
WEDNESDAY	
THURSDAY	
FRIDAY	
SATURDAY	

Eloise Laws

October Week 2

Patience - Ecclesiastes 7:8 - NL - Finishing is better than starting. Patience is better than pride.

SUNDAY	
MONDAY	
TUESDAY	
WEDNESDAY	
THURSDAY	
FRIDAY	
SATURDAY	

The Healing Shower

October Week 3

Patience - Ecclesiastes 7:8 - NL - Finishing is better than starting. Patience is better than pride.

SUNDAY	
MONDAY	
TUESDAY	
WEDNESDAY	
THURSDAY	
FRIDAY	
SATURDAY	

Eloise Laws

October Week 4

Patience - Ecclesiastes 7:8 - NL - Finishing is better than starting. Patience is better than pride.

SUNDAY	
MONDAY	
TUESDAY	
WEDNESDAY	
THURSDAY	
FRIDAY	
SATURDAY	

The Healing Shower

November Week 1

Love - Psalm 13:5 - NLT - But I trust in your unfailing love. I will rejoice because you have rescued me.

SUNDAY	
MONDAY	
TUESDAY	
WEDNESDAY	
THURSDAY	
FRIDAY	
SATURDAY	

Eloise Laws

November Week 2

Love - Psalm 13:5 - NLT - But I trust in your unfailing love. I will rejoice because you have rescued me.

SUNDAY	
MONDAY	
TUESDAY	
WEDNESDAY	
THURSDAY	
FRIDAY	
SATURDAY	

The Healing Shower

November Week 3

Love - Psalm 13:5 - NLT - But I trust in your unfailing love. I will rejoice because you have rescued me.

SUNDAY	
MONDAY	
TUESDAY	
WEDNESDAY	
THURSDAY	
FRIDAY	
SATURDAY	

Eloise Laws

November Week 4

Love - Psalm 13:5 - NLT - But I trust in your unfailing love. I will rejoice because you have rescued me.

SUNDAY	
MONDAY	
TUESDAY	
WEDNESDAY	
THURSDAY	
FRIDAY	
SATURDAY	

The Healing Shower

December Week 1

Victory - Exodus 15:2 - NLT - The LORD is my strength and my song; he has given me victory. This is my God, and I will praise him— my father's God, and I will exalt him!

SUNDAY	
MONDAY	
TUESDAY	
WEDNESDAY	
THURSDAY	
FRIDAY	
SATURDAY	

December Week 2

Victory - Exodus 15:2 - NLT - The LORD is my strength and my song; he has given me victory. This is my God, and I will praise him— my father's God, and I will exalt him!

SUNDAY	
MONDAY	
TUESDAY	
WEDNESDAY	
THURSDAY	
FRIDAY	
SATURDAY	

The Healing Shower

December Week 3

Victory - Exodus 15:2 - NLT - The LORD is my strength and my song; he has given me victory. This is my God, and I will praise him— my father's God, and I will exalt him!

SUNDAY	
MONDAY	
TUESDAY	
WEDNESDAY	
THURSDAY	
FRIDAY	
SATURDAY	

December Week 4

Victory - Exodus 15:2 - NLT - The LORD is my strength and my song; he has given me victory. This is my God, and I will praise him— my father's God, and I will exalt him!

SUNDAY	
MONDAY	
TUESDAY	
WEDNESDAY	
THURSDAY	
FRIDAY	
SATURDAY	

Important Documents

(The following documents are for the State of California only. Please check your local state offices for appropriate documents.)

Eloise Laws

APPENDIX 1 – Power of Attorney Forms (California)

CALIFORNIA GENERAL DURABLE POWER OF ATTORNEY

THE POWERS YOU GRANT BELOW ARE EFFECTIVE EVEN IF YOU BECOME DISABLED OR INCOMPETENT

CAUTION: A DURABLE POWER OF ATTORNEY IS AN IMPORTANT LEGAL DOCUMENT. BY SIGNING THE DURABLE POWER OF ATTORNEY, YOU ARE AUTHORIZING ANOTHER PERSON TO ACT FOR YOU, THE PRINCIPAL. BEFORE YOU SIGN THIS DURABLE POWER OF ATTORNEY, YOU SHOULD KNOW THESE IMPORTANT FACTS: YOUR AGENT (ATTORNEY-IN-FACT) HAS NO DUTY TO ACT UNLESS YOU AND YOUR AGENT AGREE OTHERWISE IN WRITING. THIS DOCUMENT GIVES YOUR AGENT THE POWERS TO MANAGE, DISPOSE OF, SELL, AND CONVEY YOUR REAL AND PERSONAL PROPERTY, AND TO USE YOUR PROPERTY AS SECURITY IF YOUR AGENT BORROWS MONEY ON YOUR BEHALF. THIS DOCUMENT DOES NOT GIVE YOUR AGENT THE POWER TO ACCEPT OR RECEIVE ANY OF YOUR PROPERTY, IN TRUST OR OTHERWISE, AS A GIFT, UNLESS YOU SPECIFICALLY AUTHORIZE THE AGENT TO ACCEPT OR RECEIVE A GIFT. YOUR AGENT WILL HAVE THE RIGHT TO RECEIVE REASONABLE PAYMENT FOR SERVICES PROVIDED UNDER THIS DURABLE POWER OF ATTORNEY UNLESS YOU PROVIDE OTHERWISE IN THIS POWER OF ATTORNEY. THE POWERS YOU GIVE YOUR AGENT WILL CONTINUE TO EXIST FOR YOUR ENTIRE LIFETIME, UNLESS YOU STATE THAT THE DURABLE POWER OF ATTORNEY WILL LAST FOR A SHORTER PERIOD OF TIME OR UNLESS YOU OTHERWISE TERMINATE THE DURABLE POWER OF ATTORNEY.

THE POWERS YOU GIVE YOUR AGENT IN THIS DURABLE POWER OF ATTORNEY WILL CONTINUE TO EXIST EVEN IF YOU CAN NO LONGER MAKE YOUR OWN DECISIONS RESPECTING THE MANAGEMENT OF YOUR PROPERTY. YOU CAN AMEND OR CHANGE THIS DURABLE POWER OF ATTORNEY ONLY BY EXECUTING A NEW DURABLE POWER OF ATTORNEY OR BY EXECUTING AN AMENDMENT THROUGH THE SAME FORMALITIES AS AN ORIGINAL. YOU HAVE THE RIGHT TO REVOKE OR TERMINATE THIS DURABLE POWER OF ATTORNEY AT ANY TIME, SO LONG AS YOU ARE COMPETENT.

THIS DURABLE POWER OF ATTORNEY MUST BE DATED AND MUST BE ACKNOWLEDGED BEFORE A NOTARY PUBLIC OR SIGNED BY TWO WITNESSES. IF IT IS SIGNED BY TWO WITNESSES, THEY MUST WITNESS EITHER (1) THE SIGNING OF THE POWER OF ATTORNEY OR (2) THE PRINCIPAL'S SIGNING OR ACKNOWLEDGMENT OF HIS OR HER SIGNATURE. A DURABLE POWER OF ATTORNEY THAT MAY AFFECT REAL PROPERTY SHOULD BE ACKNOWLEDGED BEFORE A NOTARY PUBLIC SO THAT IT MAY EASILY BE RECORDED.

YOU SHOULD READ THIS DURABLE POWER OF ATTORNEY CAREFULLY. WHEN EFFECTIVE, THIS DURABLE POWER OF ATTORNEY WILL GIVE YOUR AGENT THE RIGHT TO DEAL WITH PROPERTY THAT YOU NOW HAVE OR MIGHT ACQUIRE IN THE FUTURE. THE DURABLE POWER OF ATTORNEY IS IMPORTANT TO YOU. IF YOU DO NOT UNDERSTAND THE DURABLE POWER OF ATTORNEY, OR ANY PROVISION OF IT, THEN YOU SHOULD OBTAIN THE ASSISTANCE OF AN ATTORNEY OR OTHER QUALIFIED PERSON.

NOTICE TO PERSON ACCEPTING THE APPOINTMENT AS ATTORNEY-IN-FACT BY ACTING OR AGREEING TO ACT AS THE AGENT (ATTORNEY-IN-FACT) UNDER THIS POWER OF ATTORNEY YOU ASSUME THE FIDUCIARY AND OTHER LEGAL RESPONSIBILITIES OF AN AGENT. THESE RESPONSIBILITIES INCLUDE:

1. THE LEGAL DUTY TO ACT SOLELY IN THE INTEREST OF THE PRINCIPAL AND TO AVOID CONFLICTS OF INTEREST.

2. THE LEGAL DUTY TO KEEP THE PRINCIPAL'S PROPERTY SEPARATE AND DISTINCT

The Healing Shower

FROM ANY OTHER PROPERTY OWNED OR CONTROLLED BY YOU. YOU MAY NOT TRANSFER THE PRINCIPAL'S PROPERTY TO YOURSELF WITHOUT FULL AND ADEQUATE CONSIDERATION OR ACCEPT A GIFT OF THE PRINCIPAL'S PROPERTY UNLESS THIS POWER OF ATTORNEY SPECIFICALLY AUTHORIZES YOU TO TRANSFER PROPERTY TO YOURSELF OR ACCEPT A GIFT OF THE PRINCIPAL'S PROPERTY. IF YOU TRANSFER THE PRINCIPAL'S PROPERTY TO YOURSELF WITHOUT SPECIFIC AUTHORIZATION IN THE POWER OF ATTORNEY, YOU MAY BE PROSECUTED FOR FRAUD AND/OR EMBEZZLEMENT. IF THE PRINCIPAL IS 65 YEARS OF AGE OR OLDER AT THE TIME THAT THE PROPERTY IS TRANSFERRED TO YOU WITHOUT AUTHORITY, YOU MAY ALSO BE PROSECUTED FOR ELDER ABUSE UNDER PENAL CODE SECTION 368. IN ADDITION TO CRIMINAL PROSECUTION, YOU MAY ALSO BE SUED IN CIVIL COURT. I HAVE READ THE FOREGOING NOTICE AND I UNDERSTAND THE LEGAL AND FIDUCIARY DUTIES THAT I ASSUME BY ACTING OR AGREEING TO ACT AS THE AGENT (ATTORNEY-IN-FACT) UNDER THE TERMS OF THIS POWER OF ATTORNEY.

DATE:

_____
(SIGNATURE OF AGENT)

_____
(PRINT NAME OF AGENT)

CALIFORNIA GENERAL DURABLE POWER OF ATTORNEY

THE POWERS YOU GRANT BELOW ARE EFFECTIVE EVEN IF YOU BECOME DISABLED OR INCOMPETENT

NOTICE: THE POWERS GRANTED BY THIS DOCUMENT ARE BROAD AND SWEEPING. THEY ARE EXPLAINED IN THE UNIFORM STATUTORY FORM POWER OF ATTORNEY ACT. IF YOU HAVE ANY QUESTIONS ABOUT THESE POWERS, OBTAIN COMPETENT LEGAL ADVICE. THIS DOCUMENT DOES NOT AUTHORIZE ANYONE TO MAKE MEDICAL AND OTHER HEALTH-CARE DECISIONS FOR YOU. YOU MAY REVOKE THIS POWER OF ATTORNEY IF YOU LATER WISH TO DO SO. THIS POWER OF ATTORNEY IS EFFECTIVE IMMEDIATELY AND WILL CONTINUE TO BE EFFECTIVE EVEN IF YOU BECOME DISABLED, INCAPACITATED, OR INCOMPETENT.

I _____
_____ [insert your name and address] appoint
_____ [insert the name and address of the person appointed] as my Agent (attorney-in-fact) to act for me in any lawful way with respect to the following initialed subjects:

TO GRANT ALL OF THE FOLLOWING POWERS, INITIAL THE LINE IN FRONT OF (N) AND IGNORE THE LINES IN FRONT OF THE OTHER POWERS.

TO GRANT ONE OR MORE, BUT FEWER THAN ALL, OF THE FOLLOWING POWERS, INITIAL THE LINE IN FRONT OF EACH POWER YOU ARE GRANTING.

Eloise Laws

TO WITHHOLD A POWER, DO NOT INITIAL THE LINE IN FRONT OF IT. YOU MAY, BUT NEED NOT, CROSS OUT EACH POWER WITHHELD.

Note: If you initial Item A or Item B, which follow, a notarized signature will be required on behalf of the Principal.

INITIAL

_____ **(A) Real property transactions.** To lease, sell, mortgage, purchase, exchange, and acquire, and to agree, bargain, and contract for the lease, sale, purchase, exchange, and acquisition of, and to accept, take, receive, and possess any interest in real property whatsoever, on such terms and conditions, and under such covenants, as my Agent shall deem proper; and to maintain, repair, tear down, alter, rebuild, improve manage, insure, move, rent, lease, sell, convey, subject to liens, mortgages, and security deeds, and in any way or manner deal with all or any part of any interest in real property whatsoever, including specifically, but without limitation, real property lying and being situated in the State of California, under such terms and conditions, and under such covenants, as my Agent shall deem proper and may for all deferred payments accept purchase money notes payable to me and secured by mortgages or deeds to secure debt, and may from time to time collect and cancel any of said notes, mortgages, security interests, or deeds to secure debt.

_____ **(B) Tangible personal property transactions.** To lease, sell, mortgage, purchase, exchange, and acquire, and to agree, bargain, and contract for the lease, sale, purchase, exchange, and acquisition of, and to accept, take, receive, and possess any personal property whatsoever, tangible or intangible, or interest thereto, on such terms and conditions, and under such covenants, as my Agent shall deem proper; and to maintain, repair, improve, manage, insure, rent, lease, sell, convey, subject to liens or mortgages, or to take any other security interests in said property which are recognized under the Uniform Commercial Code as adopted at that time under the laws of the State of California or any applicable state, or otherwise hypothecate (pledge), and in any way or manner deal with all or any part of any real or personal property whatsoever, tangible or intangible, or any interest therein, that I own at the time of execution or may thereafter acquire, under such terms and conditions, and under such covenants, as my Agent shall deem proper.

_____ **(C) Stock and bond transactions.** To purchase, sell, exchange, surrender, assign, redeem, vote at any meeting, or otherwise transfer any and all shares of stock, bonds, or other securities in any business, association, corporation, partnership, or other legal entity, whether private or public, now or hereafter belonging to me.

_____ **(D) Commodity and option transactions.** To organize or continue and conduct any business which term includes, without limitation, any farming, manufacturing, service, mining, retailing or other type of business operation in any form, whether as a proprietorship, joint venture, partnership, corporation, trust or other legal entity; operate, buy, sell, expand, contract, terminate or liquidate any business; direct, control, supervise, manage or participate in the operation of any business and engage, compensate and discharge business managers, employees, agents, attorneys, accountants and consultants; and, in general, exercise all powers with respect to business interests and operations which the principal could if present and under no disability.

_____ **(E) Banking and other financial institution transactions.** To make, receive, sign, endorse, execute, acknowledge, deliver and possess checks, drafts, bills of exchange, letters of credit, notes, stock certificates, withdrawal receipts and deposit instruments relating to accounts or deposits in, or certificates of deposit of banks, savings and loans, credit unions, or other institutions or associations. To pay all sums of money, at any time or times, that may hereafter be owing by me upon any account, bill of exchange, check, draft, purchase, contract, note, or trade acceptance made, executed, endorsed, accepted, and delivered by me or for me in my name, by my Agent. To borrow from time to time such sums of money as my Agent may deem proper and execute promissory notes, security deeds or agreements, financing statements, or other security instruments in such form as the lender may request and renew said notes and security instruments from time to time in whole or in part. To have free access at any time or times to any safe deposit box or vault to which I might have access.

_____ **(F) Business operating transactions.** To conduct, engage in, and otherwise transact the affairs of any and all lawful business ventures of whatever nature or kind that I may now or hereafter be involved in.

_____ **(G) Insurance and annuity transactions.** To exercise or perform any act, power, duty, right, or obligation, in regard to any contract of life, accident, health, disability, liability, or other type of insurance or any combination of insurance; and to procure new or additional contracts of insurance for me and to designate the beneficiary of same; provided, however, that my Agent cannot designate himself or herself as beneficiary of any such insurance contracts.

_____ **(H) Estate, trust, and other beneficiary transactions.** To accept, receipt for, exercise, release, reject, renounce, assign, disclaim, demand, sue for, claim and recover any legacy, bequest, devise, gift or other property interest or payment due or payable to or for the principal; assert any interest in and exercise any power over any trust, estate or property subject to fiduciary control; establish a revocable trust solely for the benefit of the principal that terminates at the death of the principal and is then distributable to the legal representative of the estate of the principal; and, in general, exercise all powers with respect to estates and trusts which the principal could exercise if present and under no disability; provided, however, that the Agent may not make or change a will and may not revoke or amend a trust revocable or amendable by the principal or require the trustee of any trust for the benefit of the principal to pay income or principal to the Agent unless specific authority to that end is given.

_____ **(I) Claims and litigation.** To commence, prosecute, discontinue, or defend all actions or other legal proceedings touching my property, real or personal, or any part thereof, or touching any matter in which I or my property, real or personal, may be in any way concerned. To defend, settle, adjust, make allowances, compound, submit to arbitration, and compromise all accounts, reckonings, claims, and demands whatsoever that now are, or hereafter shall be, pending between me and any person, firm, corporation, or other legal entity, in such manner and in all respects as my Agent shall deem proper.

_____ **(J) Personal and family maintenance.** To hire accountants, attorneys at law, consultants, clerks, physicians, nurses, agents, servants, workmen, and others and to remove them, and to appoint others in their place, and to pay and allow the persons so employed such salaries, wages, or other remunerations, as my Agent shall deem proper.

_____ **(K) Benefits from Social Security, Medicare, Medicaid, or other governmental programs, or military service.** To prepare, sign and file any claim or application for Social Security, unemployment or military service benefits; sue for, settle or abandon any claims to any benefit or assistance under any federal, state, local or foreign statute or regulation; control, deposit to any account, collect, receipt for, and take title to and hold all benefits under any Social Security, unemployment, military service or other state, federal, local or foreign statute or regulation; and, in general, exercise all powers with respect to Social Security, unemployment, military service, and governmental benefits, including but not limited to Medicare and Medicaid, which the principal could exercise if present and under no disability.

_____ **(L) Retirement plan transactions.** To contribute to, withdraw from and deposit funds in any type of retirement plan (which term includes, without limitation, any tax qualified or nonqualified pension, profit sharing, stock bonus, employee savings and other retirement plan, individual retirement account, deferred compensation plan and any other type of employee

Eloise Laws

benefit plan); select and change payment options for the principal under any retirement plan; make rollover contributions from any retirement plan to other retirement plans or individual retirement accounts; exercise all investment powers available under any type of self-directed retirement plan; and, in general, exercise all powers with respect to retirement plans and retirement plan account balances which the principal could if present and under no disability.

_____ **(M) Tax matters.** To prepare, to make elections, to execute and to file all tax, social security, unemployment insurance, and informational returns required by the laws of the United States, or of any state or subdivision thereof, or of any foreign government; to prepare, to execute, and to file all other papers and instruments which the Agent shall think to be desirable or necessary for safeguarding of me against excess or illegal taxation or against penalties imposed for claimed violation of any law or other governmental regulation; and to pay, to compromise, or to contest or to apply for refunds in connection with any taxes or assessments for which I am or may be liable.

_____ **(N) ALL OF THE POWERS LISTED ABOVE.** YOU NEED NOT INITIAL ANY OTHER LINES IF YOU INITIAL LINE (N).

SPECIAL INSTRUCTIONS:

ON THE FOLLOWING LINES YOU MAY GIVE SPECIAL INSTRUCTIONS LIMITING OR EXTENDING THE POWERS GRANTED TO YOUR AGENT.

_____

_____

_____

_____

_____

_____

THIS POWER OF ATTORNEY IS EFFECTIVE IMMEDIATELY AND WILL CONTINUE UNTIL IT IS REVOKED.

THIS POWER OF ATTORNEY SHALL BE CONSTRUED AS A GENERAL DURABLE POWER OF ATTORNEY AND SHALL CONTINUE TO BE EFFECTIVE EVEN IF I BECOME DISABLED, INCAPACITATED, OR INCOMPETENT.

(YOUR AGENT WILL HAVE AUTHORITY TO EMPLOY OTHER PERSONS AS NECESSARY TO ENABLE THE AGENT TO PROPERLY EXERCISE THE POWERS GRANTED IN THIS FORM, BUT YOUR AGENT WILL HAVE TO MAKE ALL DISCRETIONARY DECISIONS. IF YOU WANT TO GIVE YOUR AGENT THE RIGHT TO DELEGATE DISCRETIONARY DECISION-MAKING POWERS TO OTHERS, YOU SHOULD KEEP THE NEXT SENTENCE, OTHERWISE IT SHOULD BE STRICKEN.)

Authority to Delegate. My Agent shall have the right by written instrument to delegate any or all of the foregoing powers involving discretionary decision-making to any person or persons whom my Agent may select, but such delegation may be amended or revoked by any agent (including

The Healing Shower

any successor) named by me who is acting under this power of attorney at the time of reference.

(YOUR AGENT WILL BE ENTITLED TO REIMBURSEMENT FOR ALL REASONABLE EXPENSES INCURRED IN ACTING UNDER THIS POWER OF ATTORNEY. STRIKE OUT THE NEXT SENTENCE IF YOU DO NOT WANT YOUR AGENT TO ALSO BE ENTITLED TO REASONABLE COMPENSATION FOR SERVICES AS AGENT.)

Right to Compensation. My Agent shall be entitled to reasonable compensation for services rendered as agent under this power of attorney.

(IF YOU WISH TO NAME SUCCESSOR AGENTS, INSERT THE NAME(S) AND ADDRESS(ES) OF SUCH SUCCESSOR(S) IN THE FOLLOWING PARAGRAPH.)

Successor Agent. If any Agent named by me shall die, become incompetent, resign or refuse to accept the office of Agent, I name the following (each to act alone and successively, in the order named) as successor(s) to such Agent:

_____

_____

Choice of Law. THIS POWER OF ATTORNEY WILL BE GOVERNED BY THE LAWS OF THE STATE OF CALIFORNIA WITHOUT REGARD FOR CONFLICTS OF LAWS PRINCIPLES. IT WAS EXECUTED IN THE STATE OF CALIFORNIA AND IS INTENDED TO BE VALID IN ALL JURISDICTIONS OF THE UNITED STATES OF AMERICA AND ALL FOREIGN NATIONS.

I am fully informed as to all the contents of this form and understand the full import of this grant of powers to my Agent.

I agree that any third party who receives a copy of this document may act under it. Revocation of the power of attorney is not effective as to a third party until the third party learns of the revocation. I agree to indemnify the third party for any claims that arise against the third party because of reliance on this power of attorney.

Signed this _____ day of _____, 20____

_____
[Your Signature]

_____
[Your Social Security Number]

CERTIFICATE OF ACKNOWLEDGMENT OF NOTARY PUBLIC

STATE OF CALIFORNIA
COUNTY OF _____

This document was acknowledged before me on _____ [Date] by
_____ [name of principal].

Eloise Laws

[Notary Seal, if any]:

_____
(Signature of Notarial Officer)

Notary Public for the State of California

My commission expires: _____

ACKNOWLEDGMENT OF AGENT

BY ACCEPTING OR ACTING UNDER THE APPOINTMENT, THE AGENT ASSUMES THE FIDUCIARY AND OTHER LEGAL RESPONSIBILITIES OF AN AGENT.

_____
[Typed or Printed Name of Agent]

_____
[Signature of Agent]

PREPARATION STATEMENT

This document was prepared by the following individual:

_____
[Typed or Printed Name]

_____
[Signature]

The Healing Shower

APPENDIX 2 – Advance Health Care Directive Form Instructions…

ADVANCE HEALTH CARE DIRECTIVE FORM

CALIFORNIA PROBATE CODE SECTION 4700-4701

4700. The form provided in Section 4701 may, but need not, be used to create an advance health care directive. The other sections of this division govern the effect of the form or any other writing used to create an advance health care directive. An individual may complete or modify all or any part of the form in Section 4701.

4701. The statutory advance health care directive form is as follows:
ADVANCE HEALTH CARE DIRECTIVE (California Probate Section 4701) Explanation

You have the right to give instructions about your own health care. You also have the right to name someone else to make health care decisions for you. This form lets you do either or both of these things. It also lets you express your wishes regarding donation of organs and the designation of your primary physician. If you use this form, you may complete or modify all or any part of it. You are free to use a different form.

Part 1 of this form is a power of attorney for health care. Part 1 lets you name another individual as agent to make health care decisions for you if you become incapable of making your own decisions or if you want someone else to make those decisions for you now even though you are still capable. You may also name an alternate agent to act for you if your first choice is not willing, able, or reasonably available to make decisions for you. (Your agent may not be an operator or employee of a community care facility or a residential care facility where you are receiving care, unless your agent is related to your or is a coworker.)

Unless the form you sign limits the authority of your agent, your agent may make all health care decisions for you. This form has a place for you to limit the authority of your agent. You need not limit the authority of your agent if you wish to rely on your agent for all health care decisions that may have to be made. If you choose not to limit the authority of your agent, your agent will have the right to:

(a) Consent or refuse consent to any care, treatment, service, or procedure to maintain, diagnose, or otherwise affect a physical or mental condition.
(b) Select or discharge health care providers and institutions.
(c) Approve or disapprove diagnostic tests, surgical procedures,and programs of medication.
(d) Direct the provision, withholding, or withdrawal of artificial nutrition and hydration and all other forms of health care,including cardiopulmonary resuscitation.
(e) Make anatomical gifts, authorize an autopsy, and direct disposition of remains.

Part 2 of this form lets you give specific instructions about any aspect of your health care, whether or not you appoint an agent.Choices are provided for you to express your wishes regarding the provision, withholding, or withdrawal of treatment to keep you alive,as well as the provision of pain relief. Space is also provided for you to add to the choices you have made or for you to write out any additional wishes. If you are satisfied to allow your agent to determine what is best for you in making end-of-life decisions, you need not fill out Part 2 of this form.

Part 3 of this form lets you express an intention to donate your bodily organs and tissues following your death.
Part 4 of this form lets you designate a physician to have primary responsibility for your health care.

After completing this form, sign and date the form at the end.The form must be signed by two qualified witnesses or acknowledged before a notary public. Give a copy of the signed and completed form to your physician, to any other health care providers you may have,to any health care institution at which you are receiving care, and to any health care agents you have named. You should talk to the person you have named as agent to make sure that he or she understands your wishes and is willing to take the responsibility.

You have the right to revoke this advance health care directive or replace this form at any time.

PART 1
POWER OF ATTORNEY FOR HEALTH CARE

(1.1) DESIGNATION OF AGENT: I designate the following individual as my agent to make health care decisions for me:

_____
(name of individual you choose as agent)

_____ _____ _____ _____
(address)   (city)   (state)   (ZIP Code)

_____ _____
(home phone)   (work phone)

Eloise Laws

ADVANCE HEALTH CARE DIRECTIVE FORM

OPTIONAL: If I revoke my agent's authority or if my agent is not willing, able, or reasonably available to make a health care decision for me, I designate as my first alternate agent:

_____

(name of individual you choose as first alternate agent)

_____

(address) (city) (state) (ZIP Code)

_____

(home phone) (work phone)

OPTIONAL: If I revoke the authority of my agent and first alternate agent or if neither is willing, able, or reasonably available to make a health care decision for me, I designate as my second alternate agent:

_____

(name of individual you choose as second alternate agent)

_____

(address) (city) (state) (ZIP Code)

_____

(home phone) (work phone)

(1.2) AGENT'S AUTHORITY: My agent is authorized to make all health care decisions for me, including decisions to provide, withhold, or withdraw artificial nutrition and hydration and all other forms of health care to keep me alive, except as I state here:

_____

_____

(Add additional sheets if needed.)

(1.3) WHEN AGENT'S AUTHORITY BECOMES EFFECTIVE: My agent's authority becomes effective when my primary physician determines that I am unable to make my own health care decisions unless I mark the following box.
If I mark this box ( ), my agent's authority to make health care decisions for me takes effect immediately.

(1.4) AGENT'S OBLIGATION: My agent shall make health care decisions for me in accordance with this power of attorney for health care, any instructions I give in Part 2 of this form, and my other wishes to the extent known to my agent. To the extent my wishes are unknown, my agent shall make health care decisions for me in accordance with what my agent determines to be in my best interest. In determining my best interest, my agent shall consider my personal values to the extent known to my agent.

(1.5) AGENT'S POSTDEATH AUTHORITY: My agent is authorized to make anatomical gifts, authorize an autopsy, and direct disposition of my remains, except as I state here or in Part 3 of this form:

_____

_____

(Add additional sheets if needed.)

The Healing Shower

ADVANCE HEALTH CARE DIRECTIVE FORM

(1.6) NOMINATION OF CONSERVATOR: If a conservator of my person needs to be appointed for me by a court, I nominate the agent designated in this form. If that agent is not willing, able, or reasonably available to act as conservator, I nominate the alternate agents whom I have named, in the order designated.

PART 2
INSTRUCTIONS FOR HEALTH CARE

If you fill out this part of the form, you may strike any wording you do not want.

(2.1) END-OF-LIFE DECISIONS: I direct that my health care providers and others involved in my care provide, withhold, or withdraw treatment in accordance with the choice I have marked below:

☐ (a) Choice Not to Prolong Life

I do not want my life to be prolonged if (1) I have an incurable and irreversible condition that will result in my death within a relatively short time, (2) I become unconscious and, to a reasonable degree of medical certainty, I will not regain consciousness, or (3) the likely risks and burdens of treatment would outweigh the expected benefits, OR

☐ (b) Choice to Prolong Life

I want my life to be prolonged as long as possible within the limits of generally accepted health care standards.

(2.2) RELIEF FROM PAIN: Except as I state in the following space, I direct that treatment for alleviation of pain or discomfort be provided at all times, even if it hastens my death:

_____

_____

(Add additional sheets if needed.)

(2.3) OTHER WISHES: (If you do not agree with any of the optional choices above and wish to write your own, or if you wish to add to the instructions you have given above, you may do so here.) I direct that:

_____

_____

(Add additional sheets if needed.)

PART 3
DONATION OF ORGANS AT DEATH
(OPTIONAL)

(3.1) Upon my death (mark applicable box):

☐ (a) I give any needed organs, tissues, or parts, OR

☐ (b) I give the following organs, tissues, or parts only.

_____

☐ (c) My gift is for the following purposes (strike any of the following you do not want):

(1) Transplant
(2) Therapy
(3) Research
(4) Education

Eloise Laws

ADVANCE HEALTH CARE DIRECTIVE FORM

PART 4
PRIMARY PHYSICIAN
(OPTIONAL)

(4.1) I designate the following physician as my primary physician:

_____
(name of physician)

_____ _____ _____ _____
(address)   (city)   (state) (ZIP Code)

_____
(phone)

OPTIONAL: If the physician I have designated above is not willing, able, or reasonably available to act as my primary physician, I designate the following physician as my primary physician:

_____
(name of physician)

_____ _____ _____ _____
(address)   (city)   (state) (ZIP Code)

_____
(phone)

PART 5

(5.1) EFFECT OF COPY: A copy of this form has the same effect as the original.

(5.2) SIGNATURE: Sign and date the form here:

_____
(print your name)

_____ _____
(sign your name)   (date)

_____ _____ _____ _____
(address)   (city)   (state) (ZIP Code)

(5.3) STATEMENT OF WITNESSES: I declare under penalty of perjury under the laws of California (1) that the individual who signed or acknowledged this advance health care directive is personally known to me, or that the individual's identity was proven to me by convincing evidence (2) that the individual signed or acknowledged this advance directive in my presence, (3) that the individual appears to be of sound mind and under no duress, fraud, or undue influence, (4) that I am not a person appointed as agent by this advance directive, and (5) that I am not the individual's health care provider, an employee of the individual's health care provider, the operator of a community care facility, an employee of an operator of a community care facility, the operator of a residential care facility for the elderly, nor an employee of an operator of a residential care facility for the elderly.

First witness   Second witness

_____   _____
(print name)   (print name)

124

The Healing Shower

ADVANCE HEALTH CARE DIRECTIVE FORM

_____   _____
(address)   (address)

_____ _____   _____ _____
(city)   (state)   (city)   (state)

_____   _____
(signature of witness)   (signature of witness)

_____   _____
(date)   (date)

(5.4) ADDITIONAL STATEMENT OF WITNESSES: At least one of the above witnesses must also sign the following declaration:

I further declare under penalty of perjury under the laws of California that I am not related to the individual executing this advance health care directive by blood, marriage, or adoption, and to the best of my knowledge, I am not entitled to any part of the individual's estate upon his or her death under a will now existing or by operation of law.

_____   _____
(signature of witness)   (signature of witness)

PART 6
SPECIAL WITNESS REQUIREMENT

(6.1) The following statement is required only if you are a patient in a skilled nursing facility--a health care facility that provides the following basic services: skilled nursing care and supportive care to patients whose primary need is for availability of skilled nursing care on an extended basis. The patient advocate or ombudsman must sign the following statement:

STATEMENT OF PATIENT ADVOCATE OR OMBUDSMAN

I declare under penalty of perjury under the laws of California that I am a patient advocate or ombudsman as designated by the State Department of Aging and that I am serving as a witness as required by Section 4675 of the Probate Code.

_____
(print your name)

_____   _____
(sign your name)   (date)

_____ _____ _____ _____
(address)   (city)   (state)   (ZIP Code)

Eloise Laws

APPENDIX 3 – Advance Health Care Directive Form

Advance Health Care Directive Form Instructions

You have the right to give instructions about your own health care.

You also have the right to name someone else to make health care decisions for you.

The Advance Health Care Directive form lets you do one or both of these things. It also lets you write down your wishes about donation of organs and the selection of your primary physician. If you use the form, you may complete or change any part of it or all of it. You are free to use a different form.

INSTRUCTIONS

Part 1: Power of Attorney

Part 1 lets you:
- **name** another person as **agent** to make health care decisions for you if you are unable to make your own decisions. You can also have your agent make decisions for you right away, even if you are still able to make your own decisions.
- also name an **alternate agent** to act for you if your first choice is not willing, able or reasonably available to make decisions for you.

Your **agent** may not be:
- an operator or employee of a community care facility or a residential care facility where you are receiving care.
- your supervising health care provider (the doctor managing your care)
- an employee of the health care institution where you are receiving care, unless your agent is related to you or is a coworker.

Your **agent** may make all health care decisions for you, <u>unless</u> you limit the authority of your agent. You do not need to limit the authority of your agent.

<u>If you want to limit the authority</u> of your agent the form includes a place where you can limit the authority of your agent.

<u>If you choose not to limit</u> the authority of your agent, your agent will have the right to:
- Consent or refuse consent to any care, treatment, service, or procedure to maintain, diagnose, or otherwise affect a physical or mental condition.
- Choose or discharge health care providers (i.e. choose a doctor for you) and institutions.
- Agree or disagree to diagnostic tests, surgical procedures, and medication plans.
- Agree or disagree with providing, withholding, or withdrawal of artificial feeding and fluids and all other forms of health care, including cardiopulmonary resuscitation (CPR).
- After your death make anatomical gifts (donate organs/tissues), authorize an autopsy, and make decisions about what will be done with your body.

Part 2: Instructions for Health Care

You can give specific instructions about any aspect of your health care, whether or not you appoint an agent.

There are choices provided on the form to help you write down your wishes regarding providing, withholding or withdrawal of treatment to keep you alive.

You can also add to the choices you have made or write out any additional wishes.

You do not need to fill out part 2 of this form if you want to allow your agent to make any decisions about your health care that he/she believes best for you without adding your specific instructions.

PS-X-MHS-442 (Rev. 3-04)   MPS/pmd

The Healing Shower

Part 3: Donation of Organs

You can write down your wishes about donating your bodily organs and tissues following your death.

Part 4: Primary Physician

You can select a physician to have primary or main responsibility for your health care.

Part 5: Signature and Witnesses
After completing the form, **sign and date it** in the section provided.

The form must be signed **by two qualified witnesses** (see the statements of the witnesses included in the form) **or** acknowledged before a notary public. **A notary is not required if the form is signed by two witnesses. The wittnesses must sign the form on the same date it is signed by the person making the Advance Directive.**

See part 6 of the form if you are a patient in a skilled nursing facility.

Part 6: Special Witness Requirement

A Patient Advocate or Ombudsman must witness the form *if you are a patient in a skilled nursing facility* (a health care facility that provides skilled nursing care and supportive care to patients). See Part 6 of the form.

You have the right to change or revoke your Advance Health Care Directive at any time

---

If you have questions about completing the Advance Directive in the hospital, please ask to speak to a Chaplain or Social Worker.

We ask that you
complete this form in English
so your caregivers can understand your directions.

127

Eloise Laws

Advance Health Care Directive

Name_____

Date_____

You have the right to give instructions about your own health care. You also have the right to name someone else to make health care decisions for you. This form also lets you write down your wishes regarding donation of organs and the designation of your primary physician. If you use this form, you may complete or change all or any part of it. You are free to use a different form.

You have the right to change or revoke this advance health care directive at any time.

Part 1 — Power of Attorney for Health Care

(1.1) DESIGNATION OF AGENT: I designate the following individual as my agent to make health care decisions for me:

Name of individual you choose as agent:_____

Relationship_____

Address: _____

_____

Telephone numbers: (Indicate home, work, cell) _____

ALTERNATE AGENT (Optional): If I revoke my agent's authority or if my agent is not willing, able, or reasonably available to make a health care decision for me, I designate as my first alternate agent:

Name of individual you choose as alternate agent:_____

Relationship_____

Address: _____

_____

Telephone numbers: (Indicate home, work, cell) _____

SECOND ALTERNATE AGENT (optional): If I revoke the authority of my agent and first alternate agent or if neither is willing, able, or reasonably available to make a health care decision for me, I designate as my second alternate agent:

Name of individual you choose as second alternate agent: _____

Address: _____

_____

Telephone numbers: (Indicate home, work, cell) _____

The Healing Shower

(1.2) AGENT'S AUTHORITY: My agent is authorized to 1) make all health care decisions for me, including decisions to provide, withhold, or withdraw artificial nutrition and hydration and all other forms of health care to keep me alive, 2) to choose a particular physician or health care facility, and 3) to receive or consent to the release of medical information and records, except as I state here:

_____

_____

(Add additional sheets if needed.)

(1.3) WHEN AGENT'S AUTHORITY BECOMES EFFECTIVE: My agent's authority becomes effective when my primary physician determines that I am unable to make my own health care decisions unless I initial the following line.

If I initial this line, my agent's authority to make health care decisions for me takes effect immediately. ____

(1.4) AGENT'S OBLIGATION: My agent shall make health care decisions for me in accordance with this power of attorney for health care, any instructions I give in Part 2 of this form, and my other wishes to the extent known to my agent. To the extent my wishes are unknown, my agent shall make health care decisions for me in accordance with what my agent determines to be my best interest. In determining my best interest, my agent shall consider my personal values to the extent known to my agent.

(1.5) AGENT'S POST DEATH AUTHORITY: My agent is authorized to make anatomical gifts, authorize an autopsy, and direct disposition of my remains, except as I state here or in Part 3 of this form:

_____

_____

(Add additional sheets if needed.)

(1.6) NOMINATION OF CONSERVATOR: If a conservator of my person needs to be appointed for me by a court, I nominate the agent designated in this form. If that agent is not willing, able, or reasonably available to act as conservator, I nominate the alternate agents whom I have named. ____ (initial here)

Part 2 — Instructions for Health Care

If you fill out this part of the form, you may strike out any wording you do not want.

(2.1) **END-OF-LIFE DECISIONS**: I direct my health care providers and others involved in my care to provide, withhold, or withdraw treatment in accordance with the choice I have marked below:

☐ a) Choice Not To Prolong
I do not want my life to be prolonged if the likely risks and burdens of treatment would outweigh the expected benefits, or if I become unconscious and, to a realistic degree of medical certainty, I will not regain consciousness, or if I have an incurable and irreversible condition that will result in my death in a relatively short time.
Or
☐ b) Choice To Prolong
I want my life to be prolonged as long as possible within the limits of generally accepted medical treatment standards.

Eloise Laws

(2.2) OTHER WISHES: If you have different or more specific instructions other than those marked above, such as: what you consider a reasonable quality of life, treatments you would consider burdensome or unacceptable, write them here.

_____
_____
_____
_____

Add additional sheets if needed.)

Part 3 — Donation of Organs at Death (Optional)

(3.1) Upon my death (mark applicable box):
- ☐ I give any needed organs, tissues, or parts
- ☐ I give the following organs, tissues or parts only:_____
- ☐ I do not wish to donate organs, tissues or parts.

My gift is for the following purposes (strike out any of the following you do not want):
    Transplant   Therapy   Research   Education

Part 4 — Primary Physician (Optional)

(4.1) I designate the following physician as my primary physician:
Name of Physician:_____
Address: _____
_____
Telephone: _____

Part 5 — Signature

(5.1) EFFECT OF A COPY: A copy of this form has the same effect as the original.

(5.2) SIGNATURE: Sign name: _____ Date: _____

(5.3) STATEMENT OF WITNESSES: I declare under penalty of perjury under the laws of California (1) that the individual who signed or acknowledged this advance health care directive is personally known to me, or that the individual's identity was proven to me by convincing evidence (2) that the individual signed or acknowledged this advance directive in my presence (3) that the individual appears to be of sound mind and under no duress, fraud, or undue influence, (4) that I am not a person appointed as agent by this advance directive, and (5) that I am not the individual's health care provider, an employee of the individual's health care provider, the operator of a community care facility, an employee of an operator of a community care facility, the operator of a residential care facility for the elderly nor an employee of an operator of a residential care facility for the elderly.

The Healing Shower

FIRST WITNESS
Print Name: _____
Address: _____
Signature of Witness: _____ Date: _____
SECOND WITNESS
Print Name: _____
Address: _____
Signature of Witness: _____ Date: _____

(5.4) ADDITIONAL STATEMENT OF WITNESSES: At least one of the above witnesses must also sign the following declaration:
I further declare under penalty of perjury under the laws of California that I am not related to the individual executing this advance directive by blood, marriage, or adoption, and to the best of my knowledge, I am not entitled to any part of the individual's estate on his or her death under a will now existing or by operation of law.

Signature of Witness: _____

Signature of Witness: _____

Part 6 — Special Witness Requirement if in a Skilled Nursing Facility

(6.1) The patient advocate or ombudsman must sign the following statement:
STATEMENT OF PATIENT ADVOCATE OF OMBUDSMAN
I declare under penalty of perjury under the laws of California that I am a patient advocate or ombudsman as designated by the State Department of Aging and that I am serving as a witness as required by section 4675 of the Probate Code:

Print Name: _____ Signature: _____
Address: _____ Date: _____

Certificate of Acknowledgement of Notary Public (Not required if signed by two witnesses)
State of California, County of _____ On this _____ day of _____ , _____ , before me, the undersigned, a Notary Public in and for said State, personally appeared _____ , personally known to me or proved to me on the basis of satisfactory evidence to be the person whose name is subscribed to the within instrument, and acknowledged
to me that he/she executed it.

WITNESS my hand an official seal.   Seal

Signature_____

PS-X-MHS-842 (Rev 2-04) Page 4 of 4 MPS/PMD

www.ingramcontent.com/pod-product-compliance
Lightning Source LLC
Chambersburg PA
CBHW070812100426
42742CB00012B/2337